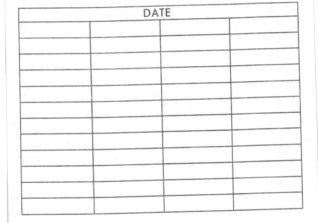

DATE			

Immunity
and
Survival

Immunity
and
Survival

Keys to Immune System Health

Sylvia S. Greenberg, Ph.D.
Long Island University, C. W. Post Campus
Brookville, New York

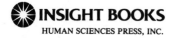

INSIGHT BOOKS
HUMAN SCIENCES PRESS, INC.

Copyright© 1989 by Human Sciences Press, Inc.
A Subsidiary of Plenum Publishing Corporation
233 Spring Street, New York, N.Y. 10013

An Insight Book

Printed in the United States of America

Library of Congress Cataloging in Publication Data

Greenberg, Sylvia S.
    Immunity and survival : keys to immune system health / Sylvia S.
Greenberg.
      p. cm.
    Includes index.
    ISBN 0-89885-435-0
    1. Immunology—Popular works. 2. Immunity. 3. Immunologic
diseases. I. Title.
QR181.7.G74 1989   88-8076
616.07'9—dc19   CIP

To my husband, Arthur, and children, Harly and Pietra, who tolerated my frequent absences from family life during the creation of this book. Their encouragement and support are deeply appreciated.

Contents

Acknowledgments

I wish to thank Dr. Ellen Duffy, Assistant Dean, School of Health Professions, Long Island University, C. W. Post Campus, and formerly of Sloan-Kettering Institute for Cancer Research, for reading the manuscript with the critical eye of an immunologist.

I am also indebted to Mr. William Lubin, a professional draftsman and artist, who contributed his talents to transform my rough figures and drawings into publishable art. In addition, as Bill came through a recent illness, he posed many questions relating to his recuperation and immunological health. He was a significant inspiration for writing this book. Since Bill displayed an urgent need to know, and was so very thankful for receiving answers, I felt that others, in similar predicaments, might benefit from the information. I hope my efforts will prove worthwhile, and will help, even a little bit.

Finally, I owe a special thanks to my husband, Dr. Arthur Greenberg, whose assistance was so essential to the accomplishment of this task. He took time from a busy practice to pitch in with the typing and editing of the manuscript.

Introduction

Evolution strives for fitness. Throughout eons of time, it has been demonstrated that the fittest survive. Using the forces of selection, evolution has enabled man to evolve with a sophisticated immune system, which facilitates his survival. The function of this system is defense. It allows us to cope with a hostile environment, which is filled with agents of disease and their deadly toxins. These pathogens need to sponge on us to prevail, and we must defend ourselves against them. Consequently, there is an ongoing struggle between them and us. Our defense system must be on the alert at all times.

The natural resistance, which is part of our heritage, is not rigidly fixed, but can be modified by many variables. Like muscles which must be cared for to stay firm and resilient, so the immune system must be maintained for best results. Knowing how to support and protect it depends on understanding the mechanics of the system. Awareness of the raw materials it needs, how it utilizes them to fulfill its function, and being informed about behavioral risks for diseases should lead to a way of life that permits the immune system to realize its full potential. By avoiding its deterrents, it is possible to intervene to prevent an illness, or to stymie its progression. An enlightened individual can reduce his vulnerability and help to improve his odds against the ubiquitous antagonists.

The immune system is at the heart of our well-being. It is involved not only with protection and recovery from disease, but it can also be the culprit in certain illnesses. It is relevant to so many areas of medicine that scientists from numerous specialties are devoting their time to the study of the body's defenses. New data is constantly being reported; so knowledge about the immune system is accumulating rapidly. There is an explosion of information, which needs to be shared with all who care about their health.

It is the purpose of *Immunity and Survival: Keys to Immune System Health* to coordinate the scientific findings about a complicated subject, and translate them into readable English. It will enable a lay audience to benefit from technical reports, which can serve as a guide for health behavior. Health knowledge can influence life-style to promote well-being and prevent disease. In order to maintain interest, an attempt was made to keep all chapters clear and succinct.

It is hoped that the book will reach those people who have a nonchalant, apathetic attitude about their health. Such individuals feel that health is the professionals' sphere. "Let my physician worry about it," they say. But what about physicians who are too busy to use those precious minutes for explanations, who assume a paternalistic attitude, who are oriented mainly towards their own specialties, and who do not emphasize prevention? Blind reverence is old-fashioned. It is smart to be able to become involved, and take an active role in decisions about your own well-being.

This book can also meet the needs of older health professionals, whose training predates the recent advances in immunology. It can serve as a quick review. Almost all areas of medicine and its allied fields are becoming involved with some aspects of the defense system. Health-care providers need to have a knowledge of the terminology and basic principles of immunology to appreciate the current reports in their technical journals. The book is designed to provide an easy way to become familiar with the subject.

Individuals who suffer from chronic illnesses can benefit from becoming acquainted with the immune system. It is always a terrible shock when you first discover you have a disease. If that isn't enough, the shock can be compounded by lack of information about what is happening within your body. Understanding the mechanism of the illness, and how it is being fought, may alleviate some of the depression that is always associated with it. Knowledge is capable of reducing the fear, anger, and pessimism that are usually brought on by a new affliction. Such negative emotions are all damaging to good immune function, at a time when it is sorely needed. In addition, being overwhelmed and emotionally drained are the perfect prerequisites for falling prey to the dispensers of "alternative therapies."

An appreciation of the underlying processes of a disease, and the interplay of factors that sustain it, can assist you in making informed decisions. It helps to be knowledgeable about the special triggering elements that may lead to setbacks, so they may be avoided. Compliance to a treatment is easier when based on understanding, rather than on blind faith or hearsay. Above all, knowledge should enable you to cope, as you channel your resources where they can do the most good. It can't hurt to know, but what you don't know *can* hurt you.

Immunology is both an old and new science. Early successes, using the techniques of immunology, involved the prevention of numerous infectious diseases that had always plagued mankind. There are reports from the beginnings of recorded history of many different diseases that ran rampant all over the world, killing thousands of people. Vaccination was the first preventive immunological strategy to be used. Even today, it is still considered to be one of the foremost discoveries in all of medicine. Successful vaccinations have protected us against so many catastrophic illnesses that the technique has earned the epithet, "the savior of mankind." The hope is that similar concepts of immunity can be utilized for the conquest of today's dread diseases, such as cancer and AIDS.

The new immunology is relatively young. It started in the late 1950s, and has resulted from findings about the cells that orchestrate the immune response, as well as the products they produce. The ability to intervene in many diseases depends on understanding the interactions between the various cell types that make up the defense system. Many practical advances in medicine are based upon this knowledge. It has been a strong factor in successes with organ transplants, treatments for allergies or hypersensitivities, and in alleviating some autoimmune diseases, where the immune system turns against parts of its own body.

Mass production of the secretions of immune cells by means of the new biotechnologies of genetic engineering are making possible novel experimental therapies for cancer. These immunotherapies are fast becoming a major ray of hope for combating this dread disease. As more work is done, and our knowledge increases, there is reason to hope that they will come into clinical use. Many unsolved problems still exist, and much remains to be learned about the immune system. However, immunology is in the forefront of today's scientific advances, and its prospects are exciting. It can influence and augment the potential for a long and happy life.

Familiarity with the subject can make you media-wise. Reports that focus on medicine, and involve the defense system, are being released with increasing frequency by newspapers, magazines, radio, and television news. Medicine is becoming a subject of great interest to the public, and immunology is on the cutting edge of medical science. It is gratifying to be able to understand and evaluate the new developments which are being discussed.

Immunity and Survival: Keys to Immune System Health can make the science of immunology become part of your general knowledge. The information will enable you to make intelligent appraisals of health-related ideas and products that are constantly being promoted to the public. It will qualify you to recognize the quack and distinguish him from the sincere scientist.

The promotion of misinformation and fraud is a growing problem affecting the vulnerable. According to a government survey involving 15 areas of health, more than one-fourth of the populace was found to be using scientifically questionable treatments and products. Since the effects can be harmful, a national conference was organized by the Food and Drug Administration (FDA) to deal with the problem. For the individual, the best defense against health fraud will always be knowledge. We can feel safe as long as we are able to sort out the facts and separate them from fiction.

Influencing you to take charge of your own health is becoming a profitable business. Specialty health stores all over the country are featuring ingenious gadgets and kits to monitor various bodily functions. They are capitalizing on the pursuit of health by healthy people, since there is much that can be done to prevent an illness. However, a prerequisite is knowledge.

Individuals with health-care knowledge usually practice prevention. They exercise more, eat less, and control stressful habits. It has also been determined that they tend to seek medical advice earlier in the course of a disease than those who are not able to recognize its signs. Better outcomes, along with lower medical costs, can be expected with earlier diagnosis. Since the immune system is central to most bodily functions, understanding how it operates may enable you to shoulder more responsibility for your own health. Awareness can lead to a better quality of life.

The enthusiastic reception of my course in immunology by

students at Long Island University and New York University has prompted me to write *Immunity and Survival: Keys to Immune System Health* for the general public. There are always lively discussions in class, with numerous examples from real-life medical experiences. The students remain glued to their chairs, even after the required time. They use words like interesting, enlightening, dynamite, and very helpful. They are sincerely thankful for being made aware of the subject.

One macho football player commented, "This class has proven to be a good conversation piece. People are amazed when I tell them how their body functions to fight off disease." Some other students, who work for health professionals, have confided that their bosses were borrowing their class notes.

The strong desire to learn in the immunology class is in sharp contrast to the cynicism displayed by some of the same students in regard to other areas of learning. If immunology is so eagerly received by both undergraduate and graduate students, shouldn't it be shared with the public?

1

Organs and Cells Involved in the Immune Response

A good quality of life is everyone's aim. To attain an aspiration so worthwhile, it is necessary to have an efficient immune system. Our protective apparatus is involved in the prevention of disease and in recuperation. All foreign invaders that attempt to prey on our bodies are recognized and fought. A good immune mechanism works silently, minute by minute of every day, frequently without our being aware of the battles raging within. On the other hand, it can also be the culprit that causes disease. As long as we understand how it operates, the tremendous power of the system may be utilized for our best advantage.

This great protector is composed of many types of cells. The cells are single units, some of which are programmed to identify specific transgressors. They work as a team, assisting one another. One sets its sights on a chickenpox virus, another on a strep throat bacterium, and still another on a malaria parasite that prefers to enter a red blood cell and destroy it. In all, it is estimated that immune cells are capable of recognizing over a million different menaces that hang around out there, always ready to pounce on us. These cells of the immune system are known as lymphocytes.

If that isn't enough protection, we also have quick-acting general purpose cells that don't have to waste any time sorting out the foe. They are nonselective in taste, and try to gobble up anything foreign that enters the body. These are the scavenger cells, or phagocytes. Evolution has provided us with two lines of defense, nonselective and selective. They team up to function as first-line and back-up defenders against most of the assailants in our environment.

Alas, harm to the body can also come from within. A body cell may spontaneously change to become a cancer cell. The alert immune system is constantly on guard for anything unfamiliar, and quickly tries to reject any altered cells. It is believed that transformed cells challenge the immune system frequently during our lives, but an effective system of surveillance prevents them from developing into cancers. Shouldn't we do everything in our power to protect our great protector?

SPECIFIC IMMUNITY

Each specific lymphocyte recognizes its antagonist by means of receptors on its surface membrane. The uniqueness of receptors is determined by genes, which are the carriers of our heredity. The receptors are so finely tuned that they identify the precise chemical characteristics of adversaries, as well as their overall three-dimensional shapes. The contours of a receptor fit the matching foe just like a lock which is coupled with its key. Some immune cells produce secretions that have the same contours as the receptors, and they also lock into the intruder. They are known as antibodies. Trespassers that are recognized by the various lymphocytes include bacteria, viruses, fungi, small and large parasites, cancer cells, some chemicals, and transplants from individuals other than identical twins.

Lymphocytes are present throughout the body, in the lymph nodes, spleen, tonsils, adenoids, appendix, thymus gland, bone marrow, blood, and lymph. They reach all parts of the body as they circulate in the connecting blood and lymph vessels. (Figure 1-1).

The tiny lymph vessels pass through most organs of the body. They pick up lymphocytes and their secretions from the lymphoid organs. A variety of tissue fluids are obtained from other organs. The resulting lymph fluid is a conglomeration of proteins, lipids, hormones, and products of the immune system. The lymph is propelled through the vessels by our muscles, whenever they contract. As the small vessels reach the chest, they merge into larger vessels, the thoracic duct and right lymphatic duct. The ducts join up with the subclavian veins, emptying the lymphatic fluid into the bloodstream.

Humoral Immunity

The system of immunity which defends the body with secretions is called humoral immunity. The term humor was used by the ancient people of medieval times to describe the fluids of the body. They believed that the humors determined the character and general health of a person. Since secreted antibodies are found in bodily fluids, and they maintain health, the system came to be known as humoral immunity.

B Cells. The lymphocytes are divided into two major groups, according to their mode of action and the targets they single out. The earliest studies of lymphocytes were concerned

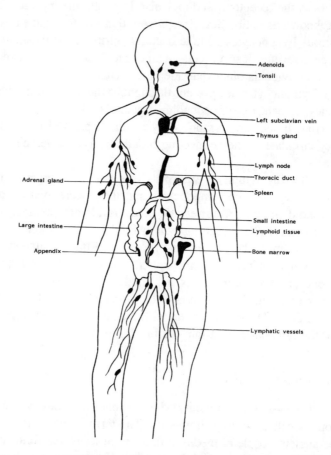

Figure 1–1.   **Organs of the human immune system. They include bone marrow, thymus gland, lymph nodes, spleen, tonsils, adenoids, lymphoid patches in intestine, appendix, and networks of lymph-carrying vessels that connect the lymphoid organs. The lymphatic vessels collect lymphocytes and antibodies. They merge into the large thoracic duct, which brings the lymphoid products to the blood stream via the subclavian veins.**

with the B cells. They are involved with the humoral system of immunity. "B" derives from bone marrow, the soft inside of our bones, which is the site of origin and the place where these cells mature. Here, each of them develops the special receptors that recognize the specific intruders. Then, they leave the bone marrow to continue the growing-up process. They enter the circulation and are carried to lymphoid organs, that are dispersed throughout the body (Figure 1–1). In their new locations, B cells wait until they can pounce on their matching foreign opponents. It is a likely place for an encounter, since these organs serve as filters to screen out unwanted substances, which are carried to them by the blood and lymph from all parts of the body. In the fury of battle, the lymphoid organs may become tender and swollen, a telltale sign of trouble within.

As soon as the receptor on a B cell becomes filled, its mission in life is consummated. It grows larger and begins to divide to form a clone of look-alikes. As an army of cells, it has greater clout against the enemy. It takes several days to increase its might.

Antibodies. Some members of the B-cell clone differentiate further into plasma cells. They function by secreting antibodies. Antibodies are large protein molecules that resemble the letter Y when viewed with the electron microscope (Figure 1–2). They circulate mainly in the lymphatic fluid and the blood. Some antibodies are able to get into other body fluids like sweat, saliva, tears, and urine. The Y-shaped molecules bear the same contours and specificity as the receptor on the B cell, which originally formed the clone. An encounter with the specific invader stimulates an interaction, whereby the trespasser becomes bound to the antibody. It is no longer free to move about or hook onto a body cell to do its damage. The whole complex then initiates further reactions that enable the body to rid itself of the spoils.

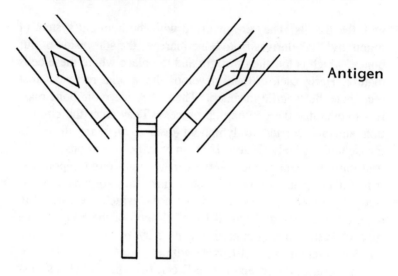

Figure 1–2. **Diagram of Y-shaped antibody. A specific antigen binding site is filled with its matching antigen.**

Any foreign invader is called an antigen. In order to become bound by an antibody, an antigen must be recognized in the fluids of the body, or when it is attached to the surface of body cells. Recognition by an antibody cannot occur if the antigen takes refuge inside a cell, because antibodies do not penetrate cellular membranes. Antibodies are part of the humoral system of immunity.

Memory Cells. Some members of the clone of large B cells, which develop after antigenic stimulation, do not go on to become plasma cells. Instead, they shrink in size and become memory cells. They are retained by the body for many years, sometimes for life. A future encounter with the same antigen that instigated the original clone leads to a secondary response. The small memory cells enlarge again, divide, and become plasma cells. The interaction of experienced memory cells with

antigen is much faster than in a primary exposure with uniniti-
ated lymphocytes. The amount of antibody produced is also
much greater. The pathogen is usually eliminated quickly in a
secondary response, before it has a chance to overwhelm the
host. The battle occurs unobtrusively, usually without any telltale symptoms. We may not even be conscious of it. With many
diseases, we can feel secure that we are immune after a first
infection, thanks to the memory cells. Persistence of memory
varies with different individuals, and it also depends on the particular antigen (Figure 1–3).

Cell-Mediated Immunity (CMI)

Another line of defense against intruders is cellular immunity. It differs from humoral immunity because no antibodies are
made. Some of the lymphocytes of CMI operate by releasing
substances which activate accessory cells, such as the nonspecific scavenger phagocytes. They are encouraged to enlarge and
make ready for the battle. Other secretions can interfere with the
replication of viruses that may have invaded body cells. Some
CMI cells attack directly and disintegrate their targets. Others
serve as assistants to many cells of the immune team, regulating
their activities. They are so important that an inadvertent reduction in their numbers can cause the entire system to collapse, as
occurs in AIDS. Some of the regulator cells function by ending
the immune reaction when it has continued on long enough.

CMI supplements humoral immunity, because it can recognize changes that occur in the interior of the cell. When the
cunning invaders hide inside, antibodies are helpless, since they
cannot traverse the membrane. There are many disease-
producing pathogens that are able to live and multiply within
body cells. These include viruses, fungi, some bacteria, and
small, one-celled protozoan parasites. CMI is also alert to spontaneous changes in normal cells, whereby they inappropriately

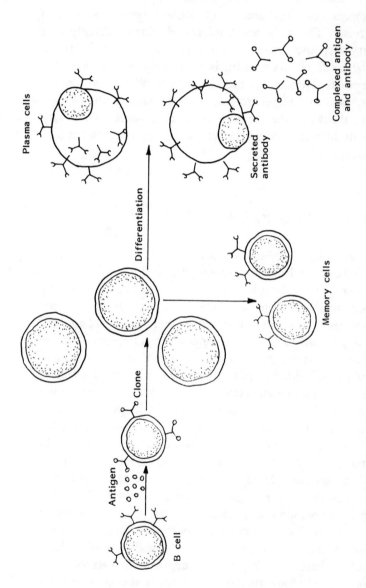

Figure 1–3. Antigen recognition by B cells leads to clone formation and differentiation into plasma cells and antigen-specific memory cells. Antibody is released from plasma cells and antigen is immobilized.

become cancer cells. Altered cells are recognized as foreign by CMI, which then works to eliminate them.

T Cells. The lymphocytes involved in cell-mediated immunity (CMI) are T cells. They originate in the bone marrow, alongside the B cells. At an early stage in their development, they leave the marrow and enter the circulation, which carries them to the thymus gland (Figure 1-1). Here they spend some time growing up. They are named "T" for their thymus gland host which nurtures them. Receptors develop on their surface membranes, enabling them to recognize specific antigens. They also differentiate into different types of lymphocytes; each has its own special way of dealing with the enemy. They can be distinguished from each other by unique surface markers, which fingerprint them.

T_K Lymphocyte. The T_K cell is a "killer" which can recognize body cells that have become tumorous. An activated T_K lymphocyte has the capacity to destroy a cancer cell by direct, intimate contact. It inflicts a "lethal hit" or the "kiss of death" (Figure 1-4) which, ideally, wipes out the potential troublemaker. T_K lymphocytes also kill cells that have become invaded by viruses. Another undertaking is rejection of transplanted organs. Here, unfortunately, T_K can't separate the good guys from the bad. When the transplant or graft comes from someone other than an identical twin, it is recognized as foreign, and is attacked. T_K goes after grafts that could be lifesaving with the same vengeance that it uses on cancer cells. In these cases, the lymphocytes must be suppressed to allow the graft to survive.

T_H Lymphocyte. T_H refers to the helper role of this lymphocyte. It interacts with other lymphocytes, both B and T, to stimulate them into action. It is a regulator of immune function, since it can amplify the activities of these cells. In fact, B cells cannot react to most antigens unless they collaborate with specific T_H cells. Part of the antigen is specific for the T_H cell and another part complexes with the B cell (Figure 1-5).

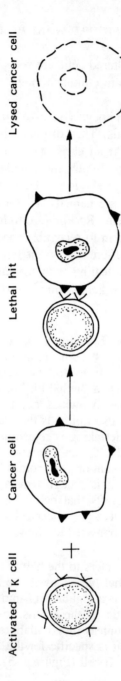

Figure 1-4. Destruction of a cancer cell by an activated killer T cell.

Activated T$_K$ cell

Cancer cell

Lethal hit

Lysed cancer cell

T_H cell   B cell

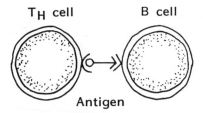

Antigen

Figure 1–5.   Model of cooperation between T_H cell and B cell. Each lymphocyte recognizes different parts of an antigen.

T_D Lymphocyte.   The T_D cell got its name because it acts in a delayed manner. An activated T_D secretes chemical mediators or signals, known as lymphokines. The mediators recruit and activate other components of the immune system to become involved in the battle against the offender. Getting others into the act takes time; so the effect of T_D cells doesn't become apparent until approximately 24 hours after the antigen entered the body. T_D lymphocytes can function against antigens which prefer to live and replicate in the interior of cells.

T_S Lymphocyte.   The T_S cell is a suppressor. It stops the immune reaction once it has proceeded far enough and has accomplished its mission. It is the control cell, which puts a halt to the battle, so it should not continue on indefinitely, perhaps to cause unnecessary and haphazard destruction. In addition, it prevents an immune attack against self-determinants, that are part of the same body. It makes sure that the immune system tolerates the body that sustains it, by suppressing aberrant lymphocytes that might want to strike out. If there is a deficiency of T_S cells, a reaction against self may occur, and autoimmune disease results. A self tissue, like a knee joint or the coating on a nerve, may be recognized as foreign, and attacked like an intruder. The results can be disastrous.

Antigen-Stimulation of T Cells.   When their stay in the thymus gland is completed, T cells enter the circulation and are carried to the various organs of the immune system (Figure 1-1). However, some of them can always be found circulating in the blood and lymph. In their various locations, they serve as surveillance cells. Each is ready to pounce on a matching antigen, which is recognized by the surface receptors. Recognition serves as a signal for the specific lymphocyte to divide. A clone of the same cell is produced, in preparation for the assault. It takes several days to assemble the defenders. Like the B cells, T lymphocytes also have memory. A second encounter with the same antigen, even many years later, is recognized faster and more efficiently than the first contact.

The humoral and cell-mediated immune systems are not independent of each other. Most immunological reactions are a cooperative effort between both systems of protection.

Nonspecific Defenders

The phagocytes are a primitive form of defense, which operate against invaders that manage to get through the protective barriers of skin and mucous membranes. They are not finicky in taste and try to engulf most intruders. Stored enzymes are always available to digest the catch, but they also make fresh poisons to attack their captives. Stimulated phagocytes can experience a respiratory burst that increases their oxygen consumption. Highly unstable, excited, toxic oxygen products are produced. They become attached to the penned-up pathogens, and an oxidative killing ensues. Then, the stored enzymes degrade them to nothingness. Phagocytes also function as the sanitation force of the body. They clean up and clear out old, used-up cells and other debris.

There are large and small phagocytes. Each type is derived from different stem cells in the bone marrow. The large cells are macrophages. The name means "big eaters." Some are fixed in the various tissues where they reside, while others move about and go wherever they are needed.

Phagocytes are the major form of protection for invertebrates, the animals without a backbone. These forms evolved early in evolution and are not endowed with the specific and discerning lymphocyte-surveillance system that we have. The more efficient back-up mechanism began with vertebrates, the animals with a backbone.

The duties of macrophages have become expanded in vertebrates. In addition to phagocytosis, they also serve as accessory cells to assist the specialized lymphocytes. By placing parts of whatever they capture on their surface membranes, they arouse the resting, susceptible lymphocytes. The prize is presented, and the tasty morsels stimulate the receptive cells into action. The response of lymphocytes when, antigens are handed to them is always superior to interactions with unshackled antigens. The macrophages also secrete many protein molecules, some of which enhance the actions of lymphocytes.

The small phagocytes are polymorphonuclear leukocytes— PMN. They are also referred to as neutrophils. PMNs are the most abundant scavengers in the blood, and usually they are the first to come to the site of an infection. They are attracted to the area by the strange chemistry of the invader. If the offender is small enough, it is engulfed and gradually killed by the products of the granules inside the PMN. If the pathogen is large and cannot be accommodated within the PMN, the granules are spilled to the outside. Granules are also pushed out of the PMN in order to digest away any damaged tissue that was hurt by the invader. During the battle, some of the PMN troops may be overcome by the toxic products produced by the enemy. When they die, they become the major component of pus.

A cell which looks like a large lymphocyte, but has none of the surface markers that are characteristic of lymphocytes, is the natural killer (NK) cell. It originates from a stem cell in the bone marrow, and is closely related to the macrophage, but it is not phagocytic. It migrates to the spleen via the blood circulation. Many NK cells are also found in the blood. They specialize in killing altered cells that have become tumor cells. Consequently, they play an important role in our natural resistance to cancer. As a first line of defense, they also recognize and deliver the death blow to cells that become infected with viruses and parasites. NK cells kill their victims by direct contact, using their toxic ingredients. They work quickly and efficiently, as soon as the culprit is recognized, and never need to waste time to become sensitized to a particular enemy. Unfortunately, the tumor-killing capacity of NK cells does not remain forever. It decreases as we grow older. As a result, tumors tend to become more prevalent with advancing years.

SUMMARY

The members of the immune team consist of nonspecific, generalized combatants and finely tuned specific specialists, one for each foe. The generalists are the first line of defense. They go into combat immediately, as soon as the enemy gains entrée, and try to gulp down anything that smells foreign to them. The nonspecific cells include the "big eaters," which are the macrophages, the smaller scavengers or polymorphonuclear leukocytes (PMN), and the natural killer (NK) cells. Each undergoes a respiratory burst, sucking in all the oxygen it can get, to make activated toxic oxygen darts. Such weapons are lethal and kill when they make contact with the target. The enemy can no longer escape. Its carcass is digested by enzymes, which are part of the arsenal of the defenders.

While the battle is raging, the specialists are getting ready. They are a more specific and more powerful back-up defense system. They are able to identify each and every enemy. This elite squad knows that it needs numbers. So, first the cells multiply to increase their ranks. The B lymphocytes grow up to become plasma cells. This takes a few days, but the generalists are there in the meantime to hold the lines. The plasma cells release antibodies that go after the enemy, wherever they can be reached. Some antibodies stay in the bloodstream and lymph, while others make their way into tissue spaces and body fluids. They grab the enemy with their contoured pincers, which are complementary to the shape of the prey. The enemy is immobilized. The antibodies are equipped with signals that flash the news of their conquest to some of the generalists. Those that are able to heed the signal come to the site to feast on the spoils.

Some of the stimulated B cells are long-lived and have good memories. They remain in the body for many years. If the same disease-causing pathogen is encountered a second time, they keep us protected or "immune" to the disease. These antibody-forming cells are responsible for humoral immunity.

The T lymphocytes also respond to the enemy by increasing their numbers. They look like B cells, but they may be differentiated by different surface markers. Some of them can get at those devilish bugs which penetrate into the inside of body cells. Altered cells, due to invaders or cancer, are identified by the surface receptors of killer cells (T_K). They adhere and kill, since they are directly toxic. Some populations of T cells produce lymphokines, which are messengers that recruit and activate other members of the immune team to come in and join the fracas.

T cells must dwell in the thymus gland during their growing-up stages. Here, they become identified as members of the cell-mediated immune system (CMI). Some of their clan work along with B cells and help regulate the humoral system of immunity. They can enhance B-cell activity with their helper cells (T_H) or suppress it with their suppressor cells (T_S). T cells also have memory, so they can act quickly and more efficiently the second time they are needed.

Fortunately, there is cooperation between the various forces of defense. Together, they put up a unified battle against assaults from the outside, as well as from within. An efficient immune team can shield us against attackers, and it contributes to the enjoyment of life.

2

The Immune System in Defense Against Disease
A Call to Action

The body can be compared to a fortress that is built for defense. It has many natural barriers to prevent invasion by infectious organisms. The outermost shield is the skin, a difficult obstacle to penetrate, when intact. In addition, the secretions from its oil glands are toxic to many of the pathogens that are always hanging around, waiting for an opening to sneak through. Hairs in the nose filter the outside air which is drawn in, so particles that might prove harmful are removed. The mucus that bathes the membranes is a barrier, too. It holds on to intruders and prevents them from making close contact with the cells. Sometimes, a few rascals manage to get by, and are sucked deep into the respiratory tract. Here, they are met by cilia, which are hairlike structures that sweep the unwelcome trespassers upward again. Another backup is a contingent of macrophages that lie in wait, ready to swallow up transgressors that happened to get past. The eye is protected by tears that wash away most trouble-makers that gain entrance. The obstinate ones that hold on are hit with enzymes that are part of the tears. The enzymes digest the intruders and erode them to nothingness.

In spite of all the outside defenses, some persistent pathogens sometimes sneak through, and make their way into the body. Then, the internal defenses take over. The scheme of events which is instigated can best be illustrated by tracking one pathogen which gained entrance. The battle with the pneumonia bacteria will be described, as it alerts the internal defense system into action.

The pneumonia bacteria, *Streptococcus pneumoniae,* is responsible for thousands of illnesses each year, with approximately 40,000 deaths in the United States, alone. It is a common disease. The hardest hit are the elderly, the chronically ill, and hospitalized patients. They account for a significant number of the deaths, and contribute heavily to the morbid statistics. Too frequently, the bacteria break through the natural external barriers of the body, and gain entrance via the membranes of the nose. The incursion alerts a good immune system into action. However, a debilitated person, with a weakened immune apparatus, may succumb to the vicious foe. Although antibiotics have increased the survival rate, they have not stemmed the tide of the disease.

The nonspecific defenses are the first to operate in the attack. PMN leukocytes are lured to the site of the invasion. They come from the bloodstream, where they normally circulate in search of prey. The unique chemical attractants of the pneumonia bacteria draw them towards the arena. When close enough, they squeeze through the blood vessel walls and stealthily creep up on the intruders. Triumphantly, some of the streptococci are devoured. Once inside the PMN, they are whacked with toxic oxygen particles and killed. Finally, the enzymes that are stored inside the PMN work to disintegrate the violators.

In a little while, reinforcements appear, which are the macrophages. They continue the mop-up operation. Some more strep are ingested and destroyed. Like good housekeepers, the "big eaters" also clean up the debris left by the battle. Body tissues that were damaged in the scuffle, as well as fallen PMN, are cleared out. The macrophages place some of the trophies of battle on their surface membranes and transport them to the lymph nodes and spleen. Here, they present their catch to lymphocytes which have the unique receptors to receive the *Strep. pneumoniae*. In a few days, the battle becomes a cooperative affair, involving the different branches of the service, specific and nonspecific. They all work against the rapidly dividing streptococcus bugs, which aim to overwhelm the host.

The B lymphocytes, which are genetically programmed to respond to *Strep. pneumoniae,* are stimulated to divide as soon as they are presented with the captives. The clone of look-alikes makes certain there is enough manpower before getting into the fight. Some of the B cells differentiate into plasma cells, the end stage of B-cell development. Others become memory cells. The plasma cells secrete unique antibodies, capable of reacting specifically with the strep. The antibodies are proteins, which are also called immunoglobulins (Ig). They get into the lymph fluid, blood, and other body secretions. Here, they form complexes with the *Strep. pneumoniae* in order to immobilize them. The bacteria can no longer move about to make their way into the lungs, the main target organ.

Five different classes of immunoglobulins are produced, each by a different member of the same clone of plasma cells. They all recognize the same strep antigen, but each is capable of acting in a different way. Each is produced in different amounts.

IMMUNOGLOBULINS (IG)

The first immunoglobulin (Ig) to be secreted is IgM. It is made in IgM-secreting plasma cells. "M" stands for macro, which describes the large size of the molecule. Its bulkiness keeps it from squeezing out of blood vessels, so it is normally not found in the tissues. It is constructed with so many pincers that it can bind five to ten similar antigens at once, depending on their size. When you visualize a policeman holding on to five scoundrels at one time, you can realize how efficient IgM is. It can be detected in the blood, in about five days after the streptococci gained entrance. It remains there for one to two months. IgM is our first line of specific antibody defense.

In about 14 days, another immunoglobulin appears in the blood, which is also specific for the same *Strep. pneumoniae.* It is IgG. There are more IgG-secreting plasma cells than IgM cells; therefore, IgG is present in the serum in larger amounts. It is the major antibody that fights the infection in later stages of the illness. IgG remains in the blood for a long time—even after the strep are defeated and the body is healed. It serves as a sentinel to protect against a rechallenge by the same invader.

If you need to know whether an infection that you recently conquered was truly due to *Strep. pneumoniae,* you can test the blood serum for the presence of specific IgM antibodies made to defend against it. Since IgM remains in the blood for only a short time, it indicates a current or recent infection. Long-lasting IgG may be present from a past bout with strep, and cannot give the information needed for distinguishing the recent disease.

IgG is a smaller molecule than IgM. It has maneuverability, and is able to squeeze in and out of blood vessels to get to the tissues, or wherever the streptococcus bug may be hiding. During pregnancy, it can also pass through the placenta, from mother to fetus. A mother's IgG protects a baby for several months after it is born. Without this supply of ready-made defenders, the baby would be vulnerable to all sorts of infections, because its own defenses take many months to develop. The newborn comes armed with all the long-lasting IgG antibodies that were made against the diseases the mother experienced. Some of her antibodies also get into breast milk, which reinforces the protection for the nursing child.

IgA is another class of immunoglobulin. It is produced by some of the plasma cells, which are members of the clone that developed from the single B cell that originally recognized the *Strep. pneumoniae*. Much of the IgA goes into body secretions, in the form of secretory IgA. It becomes part of nasal mucus, saliva, tears, sweat, and breast milk, serving as a sentry which is stationed at the entrance portals to the body. Experienced IgA can prevent a re-incursion by the same pathogen, the next time it attempts to gain entrance. The respiratory tract houses many B cells that are committed to become IgA-producing plasma cells. They protect against various respiratory insults.

IgE is normally produced by only a small number of plasma cells in the clone. Therefore, it is present in the blood in very low concentrations, and it disappears soon after being formed. Infections with bacteria like *Strep. pneumoniae* hardly raise the IgE concentration of the blood. On the other hand, large quantities of IgE can be detected in individuals infected with parasites. IgE plasma cells are stimulated into action by invading worms, such as tapeworms, roundworms, and hookworms. The secreted IgE functions by alerting its buddies to help out. These are well-equipped accessory cells, the mast cells and basophils.

Mast cells are fixed in tissues, whereas basophils circulate in the blood. The IgE attaches itself to receptors on the surface of each of these cell types. When the IgE contacts its specific antigen, it forces the shackled cells to release their stored granules, which contain several potent chemicals. Histamine is one of the important secretions. It dilates blood vessels, so more blood can come into the area, to bring in its armed might. The permeability of the vessels is also increased, allowing the large defenders as well as the parasites to move out.

IgE is made in huge amounts in allergic individuals, in response to many harmless antigens. People who are sensitive to inhaled allergens, like dust and pollen, or some food allergens, make an exaggerated amount of IgE. They suffer from the powerful effects of the mediators that are released by mast cells and basophils. The results are the uncomfortable symptoms usually associated with allergies, such as red, tearing eyes, swollen, running nose, or hives. The released histamine can also cause a contraction of smooth muscles in the airways. Air is prevented from getting into the lungs. The wheezing and gasping for breath that is associated with asthma results. IgE can be a troublemaker and a formidable foe to deal with.

IgD was discovered only recently, because it is formed in such minute amounts that detection is difficult. It appears fleetingly, and breaks down readily. Together with IgM, it serves as a receptor on the B-cell membrane. Both of these immunoglobulin molecules, on a single B cell, have unique pincers that recognize the same antigen. The B lymphpocyte recognizes the prey and locks into it by means of its IgD and IgM receptors. The joining serves as a signal for the B cell to divide and form a clone that differentiates into plasma cells. There is no other known function for IgD.

When the B-cell clone is forming, switches occur in the programming of the genes of every member. Each program dictates the production of only one of the five different immunoglobulin classes: IgM, G, A, D, or E. When they become fully differentiated plasma cells, each clone member secretes a different Ig class. The immunoglobulins are all directed against the same antigen, but each type is able to maneuver through the body in different ways.

Some of the B lymphocytes remain as memory cells, instead of differentiating into plasma cells. They live a long time after the patient has recovered, and continue to protect against future encounters with the same *Strep. pneumoniae* enemy. A second invasion, even many years later, elicits a faster and more efficient response than is possible with a primary confrontation. There is no need to take the time to sensitize the cells. They are ready and waiting. Within a few hours of a secondary confrontation, the concentration of antibody which is produced is greater than after a primary reaction. The IgG type predominates, and it holds onto its prey tenaciously. The defense system is always better prepared the second time around (Figure 2-1).

T LYMPHOCYTES

A T_H cell that is specific for *Strep. pneumoniae* is also stimulated into action by the presenting macrophage. T_H is programmed by its genes to recognize a different portion of the pneumonia bug than the B cell. It divides to form a clone in preparation for the attack. Each member of the clone then collaborates with a member of the B-cell clone, as they both hold on to different parts of the catch (Figure 1-5). This alliance enables members of the B-cell clone to switch genetic programs in order to differentiate into different plasma cells, each capable of manufacturing one of the five antibody classes. Without the help of the T_H cell, the B cell can only produce limited clones of IgM-secreting plasma cells. Production of the short-lived IgM is independent of association with the T_H cell (Figure 2-2).

After enough antibody has been produced to inactivate the *Strep. pneumoniae,* the battle must be terminated, to prevent the response from continuing on indefinitely. Evolution has provided us with several ways to stem the reaction. One of these is the specific suppressor T cell. A T_S cell, which is specific for the same *Strep. pneumoniae* that activated both the T_H and B cells, produces a factor that binds to the lymphocytes and stops their action. One of the regulators of suppressor activity is the T_H cell, itself. T_H can determine when the clone of T_S cells should be formed, and how many cells are needed. If too much T_S activity

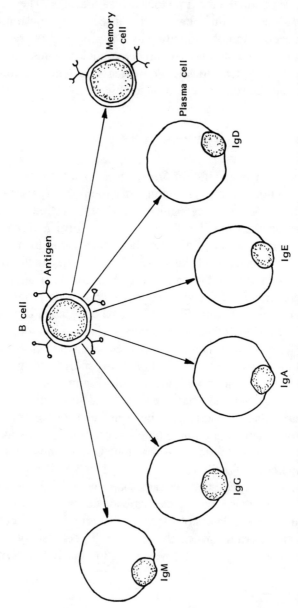

Figure 2–1. B cell differentiation in the presence of antigen results in plasma cells and memory cells. The plasma cells secrete different immunoglobulins, each of which is specific for the same antigen.

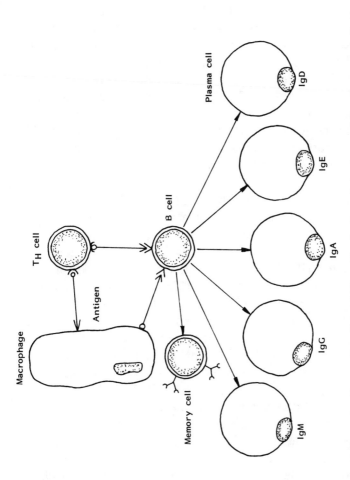

Figure 2–2. Interaction of macrophage, B cell and T_H cell. Antigen is processed by the macrophage. It activates a helper T cell which stimulates the B cell that has antigen bound on its receptors. The B cell divides to form a clone, plasma cells, and memory cells.

develops too soon, it can interfere with both the B- and T_H-cell function, and prevent an adequate immune response. The *Strep. pneumoniae* would become the declared winner. If there are too few T_S cells, a pathologic overreactivity of the B and T cells can result. They continue to function long after the *Strep. pneumoniae* are demolished, and can hurt innocent body tissues.

A normal contingent of T_S cells is one of the methods the immune system uses to hold T_H in line. T_S can prevent an aberrant immune response, which may be formed against self tissues. The correct balance of T_H to T_S lymphocytes contributes to normal tolerance of self. Autoimmune reactions are prevented.

The T_H cell may be considered to be the pivotal cell in the immune network. It busies itself with the affairs of many other cells that are reacting to the same antigen. Not only does it cooperate with B cells, and call on T suppressor cells to terminate its own activities, but it is the major producer of interleukin-2 (IL-2). This factor affects other cells of the immune team. IL-2 stimulates killer T cells to become attack cells against cancer and virally infected cells. In addition, it increases the growth and activity of natural killer (NK) cells, which also go after cancer cells and those that are invaded by viruses. IL-2 was originally called T-cell growth factor (TCGF), because it also promotes the growth of the same T_H cells that produce it. Maintaining an adequate supply of the all-important T_H cells is essential for healthy immune function (Figure 2–3).

The major response of the body to an incursion by *Strep. pneumoniae* is humoral. The transgressors are visible on the outside of cells, so antibodies can attack them. However, some of the lymphocytes that belong to the cell-mediated branch of immunity (CMI) help in the regulation of the humoral attack against the strep. The T_H and T_S lymphocytes of CMI are involved. Here, the two systems of immunity overlap.

The other CMI cells prefer to respond mainly to invaders that seek refuge inside of cells. T_D and T_K are sensitive to patho-

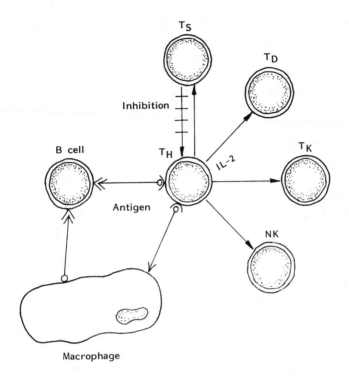

Figure 2–3. T_H **lymphocyte is the pivotal cell in the immune reaction.** → = stimulate.

gens that remain invisible to the action of antibodies. They also respond to self cells that become cancerous. With the dual system of defense, the body is able to rout out most foreign invaders, no matter where they reside.

THE ANTIGEN-ANTIBODY COMPLEX

The specific antibody that codes for *Strep. pneumoniae* identifies its quarry and combines with it. The antigen is shackled and can no longer attack. Then, the complex sends out a signal which lures nonspecific phagocytes to the spot. They rush in and gulp down the whole thing. The tasty morsels are digested with enzymes that are stored within the "big eaters" and PMNs.

If a complexing antibody belongs to the IgM or IgG class, an additional nonspecific accessory system is also mobilized to help with the destruction. This is a family of proteins, known as the complement system (C). Complement is a normal constituent of the blood. As the IgG or IgM grasps the strep with the arms of the molecule (Figure 1–2), the tail end binds to the first complement protein in the family, C_1. Binding activates C_1 to become an enzyme that has the power to activate and bind the next complement protein in the series. Like an army of tin soldiers, each knocking down the next, each complement protein in the sequence activates the next in line. As they bind to each other, the chain grows longer, until C_9 is reached. The whole reaction is called the complement cascade. The C_5 to C_9 end of the chain is the killer complex. It punctures a hole in the shackled antigen and destroys it. Now, even if the antibody lets go, the injured *Strep. pneumoniae* can do no more harm. The attached complement also escalates the phagocytic activity of the macrophages and PMNs. They are attracted to the site, and quickly mop up the carcasses. The body won the first round against *Strep. pneumoniae*.

IMMUNE COOPERATION

The successful functioning of specific B and T lymphocytes depends on the assistance of the all-purpose macrophages and PMN leukocytes, as well as the complement proteins. They all work together for the singular purpose of ridding the body of the illness. Evolution has provided us with an interacting network and back-up systems. The total reaction is necessary for good health. A failure in any part of the response means trouble.

Deficiencies in parts of the system sometimes occur. They can be inherited or acquired. Affected individuals suffer frequent infections from both the usual agents of disease, as well as from those that are rarely troublesome to others. In addition, the incidence of tumors in immunodeficient individuals is high. Normally, T lymphocytes recognize newly arising cancer cells by means of telltale markers on the outer membrane. A reaction is quickly triggered to destroy them. With an immunodeficiency, there may be no recognition response. The proliferation of the cancer cell is unimpeded, until it eventually destroys the host.

Life Cycle of the Immune System

Immune capacity varies during the different stages of life. Babies are born with an incompletely developed system of protection. They depend mainly on the mother's IgG, which passed through the placenta during the fetal stage. It fills the gap until the baby gradually develops its own capabilities. Breast milk also serves as a good source of borrowed, ready-made IgA and IgG. These immunoglobulins protect the stomach and intestine of the nursing infant.

The immune system matures gradually, reaching the height of its protective ability from late childhood to early adulthood. Measurements of the thymus gland have shown that it reaches its maximum size at puberty. Then, it gradually shrinks, retaining only about 10 percent of its weight by the age of fifty. Most of its structure becomes fibrous and fatty. The thymic hormone, thymosin, which influences the maturation of young T cells, begins to decrease in concentration in a twenty-year-old. By the age of sixty, it can no longer be detected in the blood. From these measurements, it is possible to interpret the motives of evolution. The immune system may have evolved to give maximum protection during the reproductive years. After that, you are on your own. However, the outlook is really not so gloomy, since we have thousands of memory cells from previous contacts with pathogens. They may be activated long after the thymus shrinks into oblivion.

Nevertheless, lack of immune competence is associated with aging. A recent study at the Mayo Clinic has shown that the attack rate of the viral disease, shingles, increases dramatically past age seventy. A selective decline in CMI for the shingles virus has been postulated. The elderly also have a high risk of contracting other infectious diseases and cancer. *Strep. pneumoniae* is a frequent winner in the aged.

Another affliction that may develop with advancing years is autoimmune disease. Defects can occur in immune regulation due to the loss of one cell type, such as the suppressor T cell. Without suppression of the immune response, aberrant lymphocytes that are able to recognize self tissues as antigens are allowed to function. An organ, such as the kidney, or essential nerves in the brain may be attacked. The degeneration eventually leads to organ failure and death.

The aging process involves changes in body composition and a deterioration of some physiologic functions. To what extent this is a consequence of immune senescence has not been defined. Research with immune enhancement, for the purpose of protection from disease, may eventually result in the happy side effect of delayed aging. Immunity must be a key factor in longevity, since it confers significant advantages for survival. Perhaps boosting the immune system will allow us to reach our life span potential, which has been estimated to be 115 years. In any event, immune enhancement can improve the quality of life, no matter how long it is.

Summary

An episode in the life of a pneumonia bacterium is described. It surmounts the natural barriers of the body and gains entrance. A healthy immune system is alerted into immediate action. First the PMN leukocytes and macrophages come after it. Then the B and T cells respond. The B cells are prodded to grow up fast and become plasma cells, to secrete their immunoglobulin juices. Five different classes of immunoglobulins are made. Each is capable of reacting with the same enemy, but each does the job in its own special way. All for a better killing!

IgM is the first to appear. It can capture at least five *Strep. pneumoniae* at once. Then IgG gets into the act. It hangs around for a long time, ready to pounce in case of a recurrence. Much of the IgA goes into body secretions. It guards all body openings in contact with the environment. IgE is made in minute amounts, because *Strep. pneumoniae* is not its cup of tea. IgD is a fragile fighter, which is placed on the B-cell membrane. It serves to identify the culprit. It grabs it and holds on until further help can arrive.

T_H cells, which are programmed to respond to *Strep. pneumoniae*, increase their ranks in preparation for the attack. They interact with the specific B cells, forcing them to switch immunoglobulin classes. They make certain that all five are manufactured. Variety improves efficiency. When enough is enough, T_S cells specific for the strep get into the act. They help to end the fight. The other members of the T cell population, T_D and T_K, lurk on the sidelines, waiting for their special kind of prey. They like pathogens that live and multiply inside of body cells.

The complexes, formed by immunoglobulins M and G with *Strep. pneumoniae*, call complement proteins into action. A complement cascade, which involves an intricate chain of nine proteins, is initiated. A killer complex finally punches holes in the immobilized strep. Its life is terminated. Good riddance!

Age brings about changes in the immune system. The thymus gland, especially, can reveal your age. It begins to decline after puberty. Memory cells become important in keeping the oldies going. If we could boost the immune system, and keep it functioning into old age, the fountain of youth might become reality. Eventually, techniques of immune enhancement may be able to outfox time, so nobody will grow old before four score and twenty.

3

Immune Enhancement to Control Disease

Exploiting Our Potential

The immune system of a newborn baby is naive. The infant emerges into a hostile world of pathogens with few defenses of its own. Fortunately, the dependable mother shared her IgG antibodies, through the placenta, with the fetus. Mother's prescience protects the young with her own immunological experiences.

The transfer of prefabricated antibodies from the mother gives the child a passive form of immunity. These antibodies are only temporary protectors; but they serve valiantly to fill the gap, until the baby's own defenses are developed.

Gradually, as the child is exposed to the ever-present antigens of the environment, he learns how to cope on his own. His B and T lymphocytes are actively stimulated to develop clones with memory cells. They supply a long-lasting, specific immunity.

NATURALLY ACQUIRED IMMUNITY

The ability to develop a natural immune response to pathogens has been recognized and chronicled since early times. The ancient people understood immunological memory, and realized that recovery from some illnesses protects against contracting them a second time. The body actively acquires immunity to the disease it has fought. People tried to protect their children by purposely exposing them to sick persons who had mild cases of infectious diseases. The hope was that the children would also contract mild cases, and then become immune to later encounters. This was fraught with danger, since we know now that the severity of an infection is influenced by the individual's ability to react to the agent of disease. It is determined by the strength of his immune response to the particular pathogen. If the retaliation is good, the illness is mild. With an inadequate strike back, it could be severe, since the pathogens are not well controlled, and soon enjoy the upper hand. The quality of the response depends on genetic programming for the specific antigen, nutritional status, age, and general health. It is a combination of controllable and uncontrollable factors. In addition, some pathogens mutate readily and may increase their virulence while in the body.

ARTIFICIALLY ACQUIRED IMMUNITY

A safe, scientifically controlled attempt to artificially establish immunity against an infectious disease was first undertaken by Edward Jenner in 1796. His aim was to prime the immune system while healthy, so it could successfully handle an invasion by the same bug at a later time. He studied farm workers who contracted the mild cowpox disease from cows. He noted that none of these people ever came down with smallpox, a dreaded, disfiguring, and killer disease, even though they had contact with victims. Why not deliberately inject people with the innocuous cowpox to stimulate active immunity against smallpox? Jenner's experiments were successful. The procedure came to be called vaccination, since the Latin word *vacca* means cow.

Jenner started the first vaccination against smallpox by using pus from a lesion in a dairymaid who had cowpox. He injected a healthy subject, who subsequently came down with the mild, localized cowpox disease. After a while, he inoculated the same patient with pus from the lesion of a smallpox victim. He failed to get smallpox! We know now that the virus which causes cowpox is very similar to the smallpox virus. They share many determinants in common, and the immune reaction made against one virus cross-reacts with the other. Once the body mobilized its defenses and produced memory cells against cowpox, it also became immune to smallpox.

Later, an altered form of the smallpox virus was used as the immunizing agent. It was prepared by transferring the virus through the skin of calves or rabbits. Each new habitat caused the virus to mutate, so that it changed to a less virulent form. Its major disease-producing properties were lost, but not the identity of the virus. The attenuated form served as a safe vaccine. It fooled the body into making an immune response with memory cells. Whenever the real virus was encountered, it was clobbered by the alert and experienced immune cells of the vaccinated individual. The enemy did not stand a chance. Today, many different pathogens are modified by means of heat, radiation, or chemicals to make vaccines.

Smallpox vaccination is no longer needed today, because worldwide use of the vaccine has eradicated the disease. Billions of immune systems were successfully manipulated, until we finally got rid of a virus which had plagued mankind for thousands of years. It has become an extinct species.

Vaccines for other vicious diseases are available. The continued existence of many afflictions like polio, measles, diphtheria, whooping cough, tetanus, rubella, hepatitis B, mumps, and pneumonia-related infections, can be blamed on negligence, or lack of awareness about vaccination. High cost may also be a factor.

A recent addition to the vaccine arsenal operates against the debilitating malaria parasite. It is expected that the artificially stimulated immunologic attack will eventually spare the millions of people who live in the malaria belts of the world.

Vaccinations are able to prevent epidemics before they happen. The beneficial effects on the welfare of the world's population and on its economy are astronomical. During epidemics, there are always costly hospitalizations, loss of time from work, and even deaths. Economic progress is undermined by ill health. Vaccines are cheap by comparison. Vaccination is considered to be one of the most important discoveries that has been made in the long history of medicine.

Unfortunately, there are still many infectious diseases which have eluded control by means of vaccines. The attempts to neutralize them with antibiotics and drugs can only be made after the attack. They continue to spread, and are never wiped out. In addition, the pathogens frequently develop resistance to antibiotics, and new remedies must continuously be developed. Successful vaccines are the only effective means for mass protection, and the eventual elimination of a disease.

When vaccine technology is not effective, it may be due to a variety of factors that enable a cunning, infectious organism to defy control. Some of the bugs are not immunogenic enough and do not stimulate a good antibody response. Eventually, scientists will have to find a way to bind them to carriers that modify their guise, to arouse the immune system and promote recognition. Some pathogens don't grow in the test tube, outside the body, making it difficult to obtain the quantities needed for vaccine preparation. Some viruses are adept at changing antigenic identity. The specific vaccine prepared against one form has little capability against succeeding variants. Mutations allow these viruses to always stay one step ahead of the vaccines.

An example is the influenza virus. Vaccines are available, but they must be prepared anew periodically, as variants emerge. In addition, the immunity induced by these vaccines is short-lived, because killed preparations are in use. They are not as antigenic as live vaccines. Currently, researchers are experimenting with live, mutated viruses that are capable of growing only at low temperatures. Although they fail to survive in the warmth of the lungs, they do stimulate immunity. This attenuated, live virus is being used successfully in Russia. It can be administered very comfortably as a nasal spray, which is also the natural route of entry of the virus.

The common cold has been traced to hundreds of antigenically distinct forms of the cold virus. Preparation of an effective vaccine has frustrated science for a long time, and appears to be an insurmountable task. Instead, some immunologists are now concentrating on blocking the receptor sites in the nose that are used by the virus to gain entrance into the body. They are experimenting with an antibody that is prepared against the natural human receptor. It is made in an unrelated species, which is injected with the human nasal preparation. Since the human antigen is recognized as foreign, antibody formation is stimulated. The isolated antibody is able to unite with the viral receptor sites in the nose. The entryways for the virus become blocked, and can no longer be used for attachment. The virus is turned away. By the clever manipulation of the defense system, it is hoped that the stuffy nose may someday become a harassment of the past.

Other vaccine strategies are being developed, using *parts* of a pathogen, rather than the whole organism. This is an advantage, especially when used in lieu of a live vaccine. There is always the fear that a whole, attenuated, live organism may mutate while in the body, and revert back to its original, virulent form. On the other hand, if only a key immunogenic piece of the pathogen is used, it can stimulate the formation of an antibody that will also neutralize the whole invader whenever it is encountered. Problems of toxicity can be avoided, and there may be fewer adverse reactions.

Such a strategy is being tried for mutating pathogens like the cold virus. It would be a boon to mankind if a critical part of this ever-changing pest could be found which is common to all the variants. One vaccine would then hit all.

As different tactics for vaccine preparations continue to be explored, perhaps more of our microscopic opponents will eventually succumb. After all, immunology is still a developing science, and the immune system has not been fully elucidated.

ALL-NATURAL AGENTS THAT FIGHT DISEASE

It seems logical that escalating the body's own immune system, so that it takes a more forceful role in fighting a disease, would be a superior alternative to less specific treatments with chemicals or therapy with radiation. The latter methods often cause severe side effects by harming healthy tissues along with those that are targeted. Immune enhancement, with naturally occurring body substances, is being tried experimentally in cancer and acquired immunodeficiency syndrome (AIDS). Many of the natural products can be made in large quantities by the remarkable technology of genetic engineering. The hope is that they will boost the immune system's own rejection response. The body's natural resources are finally being exploited. So far, the results have not reached theoretical expectations. However, the potential is so great that researchers are undaunted and keep trying. By manipulating the methods of administration of biological agents, and by using different combinations, the objectives of treatment may yet be realized. There is reason to believe that immunotherapy is the new hope for the treatment of many diseases.

Interferon (IF)

Interferon was one of the first body substances to show potential against viral diseases and cancer. It consists of a group of natural proteins that are produced in very small amounts by human cells. The secretions can inhibit viral multiplication, and they serve as a signal to call other cells of the immune team into action. Interferon is usually made in a virus-infected cell, and is released into the extra-cellular space. Neighboring cells that are not yet infected with the virus pick up the IF. Cells have specific receptor sites to receive it. The newly acquired protein protects these healthy cells from the spreading virus by blocking its reproduction. Interferon responds quickly to a viral infection before the specific immune response has had time to develop. It is one of our first lines of defense, which holds back the enemy until reinforcements appear.

Interferon also sparks nonspecific protector cells, like macrophages and natural killer (NK) cells to become active. Since one of the functions of these cells is to destroy tumor cells, IF serves as the go-between that is associated with antitumor activity. Indeed, the American Cancer Society chose to promote IF as a toxic agent against cancer due to its enhancing effect on NK activity. It invested $2 million in IF research, betting that it could win in the fight against cancer. So far, the investment has not totally paid off. Interferon appears to be effective in a limited number of cancers. The FDA (Federal Drug Administration) gave its approval for interferon in the treatment of hairy cell leukemia, which accounts for 2 percent of adult leukemias. It has become the treatment of choice for this cancer.

Many scientists still feel that IF is a natural weapon which has the potential to eliminate other cancers, too. It is being tried as part of a combination program, along with other biological agents for resistant cancers.

Interleukin-2 (IL-2)

IL-2 is a natural product of T_H cells. It operates by sending a message to other defense cells to proliferate and become active. It incites killer T cells and NK cells to hurry up and get into the fight. Its surrogates then attack virus-infected cells and cancer cells. IL-2 also stimulates the development of more T_H cells to provide reinforcements for the battle. It is a natural immune enhancer that can now be made in unlimited quantities by genetic engineering.

IL-2 is being tried experimentally in some terminal cancer patients to escalate immune rejection of the tumor. It is showing dramatic results against certain forms of cancer, but side effects are limiting its use.

The therapeutic approaches with IL-2 have been novel and daring. In one method, the patient's lymphocytes are removed from his blood by a process called leukophoresis. They are cultured outside the body for 3 to 4 days, in the presence of IL-2. When the cells become stirred up and activated, they are returned to the bloodstream, together with more IL-2. The aroused lymphocytes have caused cancers to shrink in some patients, but the side effects are a problem.

Another mode of treatment involves extracting the lymphocytes that are found in a tumor biopsy specimen. It is reasoned that immune cells, which are in intimate contact with the tumor, should have specificity for the tumor antigens. They are provoked in the test tube, by culturing with IL-2 for several days. After activation, the cells are returned to the patient. The treatment with IL-2 makes the lymphocytes about 100 times more toxic to the tumor than before.

Some neurosurgeons are experimenting with implants of

IL-2-treated lymphocytes directly into the tumor bed. The lymphocytes are originally obtained from the peripheral blood of the patient. After being treated with IL-2 in vitro, they are implanted at the tumor site. The method combines surgical removal of as much tumor tissue as possible, followed by IL-2 therapy. It is being used experimentally in terminal patients with brain tumors. Survival has been prolonged without serious side effects.

Tumor Necrosis Factor (TNF)

TNF is another addition to the cancer immunotherapy arsenal. Normally, it is secreted by macrophages which have become aroused. It is a protein that causes hemorrhaging within tumors, and can ultimately lead to their destruction. It is also responsible for the wasting and weight loss which typically occur in people with prolonged chronic diseases. The genes that code for the factor have been isolated, so it can be produced in therapeutically useful quantities by genetic engineering. Trials with terminal cancer patients are being conducted to boost immune might, when the disease no longer responds to conventional therapies. Regressions have been achieved when TNF is injected directly into the cancer. However, there are side effects such as fever and lowered blood pressure. TNF is enhanced by interferon.

Colony-Stimulating Factors (CSFs)

Hormones that are produced by body cells in very small quantities have been found to influence the growth and differentiation of bone marrow cells. Much exciting work is being done with these biologicals, as they are now available in plentiful amounts. The genes coding for them have been identified, so they can be manufactured on demand. The CSFs enhance body defenses by goading the stem cells of the marrow into making more cells, especially PMNs and macrophages. These are our first-line defenders against many diseases. They are being tried in bone marrow transplant patients, AIDS, and cancer.

Thymosin

A hormone from the thymus gland, thymosin, is a biological agent that is being used in experimental therapies to combat cancer, AIDS, and hereditary deficiencies (Figure 1-1). Physiologically, thymosin is involved in the differentiation of young T lymphocytes, which come from the bone marrow and settle in the thymus gland. During their sojourn here, they mature into specific classes of T cells, under the influence of the hormone. Clinically, thymosin is used for its restorative effect when immune function is suppressed. It increases the number of active T lymphocytes so they may become involved in defense. Unfortunately, the effect is not long-lasting.

Thymosin is probably one of many factors that are needed for a successful immune response. The specific contributions of all the natural agents will have to be sorted out before they can be put back together again for effective immunotherapy. Combination treatments need to mimic the response of the immune system, which normally produces all the different substances at the same time. It is hoped that regulated doses will work to inactivate cancer cells that succeeded in escaping immune controls. Our ability to manipulate the doses of natural products, which are being made available by genetic engineering, brings us a step closer to controlling our own destinies in the battle against the killer diseases.

Monoclonal Antibodies

Monoclonal antibodies have revolutionized immunology, and their impact on clinical medicine is enormous. They consist of identical antibody molecules, produced by a single look-alike clone of cells. The antibodies can be manufactured outside the body, in unlimited quantities. The Nobel prize in medicine and physiology has been awarded for the development of the technique by which the cellular manufacturing units are prepared. They are known as hybridomas.

In order to stimulate the production of the desired antibody, B lymphocytes are obtained from the spleen of a mouse which has previously been injected with the target antigen. Some of the B cells that are collected have the potential to differentiate into plasma cells that will make the needed antibody. The B cells are fused with a line of tumorous plasma cells in the test tube. They form hybrid cells or hybridomas.

Normally, B lymphocytes do not survive very long when grown outside the body. This is overcome by fusing or hybridizing them with immortal, perpetually dividing tumorous plasma cells. A line of aberrant plasma cells is used that is incapable of producing its own antibody. Fusion is accomplished with polyethylene glycol, which is antifreeze. Eternal, continuously growing hybridomas result. Each fused unit has the capacity for endless cell divisions, characteristic of the tumor cell component, and an unlimited output of the specific antibody that the B cell constituent is programmed to produce. The hybridoma has the best of both worlds. By a weeding-out process, the unique hybrid that produces the desired antibody is selected for continuous growth. Its antibodies are homogeneous, since they are produced by a clone, and the quantities are unlimited. They are used in medicine, both for diagnosis and therapy (Figure 3-1).

Monoclonal antibodies can be tailor-made to function against almost any desired antigen. For example, the unique determinants on tumor cells of cancer victims are being used as antigens. Hybridomas that make unlimited antibodies against the tumors are produced. The antibodies can be attached to radioactive chemicals and injected into the body to seek out the specific tumor cell antigens. The tagged complexes emit radiation that reveals the location of all cancer cells. Those that have spread or

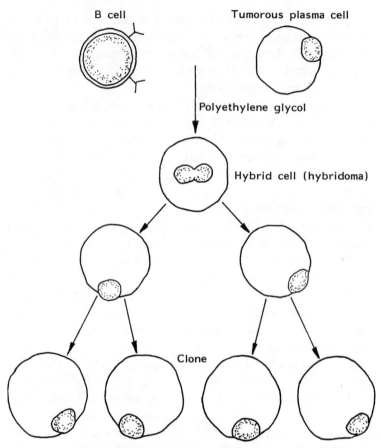

Figure 3.–1. Synthesis of monoclonal antibodies. All members of the clone produce the same antibody which is determined by the antigen-stimulated B cell.

metastasized to new locations, where they set up satellite colonies, can be identified.

Specific monoclonals that are attached to tracers can differentiate the various types of leukemias and lymphomas. Most of the cell types involved in these diseases have unique markers on their surface membranes. The matching monoclonal antibody that locks into the antigenic marker on the tumor cell identifies the exact cell type. Knowing the cell type frequently determines the type of treatment that is prescribed.

The success of a particular treatment that is being used for a cancer patient can be monitored with a monoclonal antibody specific for the tumor. If the cancer was not completely eradicated by the prescribed chemotherapy or radiation, its presence would be disclosed by the specific antibody, attached to a revealing marker.

The therapeutic potential of monoclonals in the battle against cancer is being explored. When a tumor-specific antibody is made, and then linked to a poison, the monoclonal can bring the deadly chemical directly to the tumor cell. Like a magic bullet, it can deliver its deadly cargo, accurately aimed at the cancer, without involving other tissues. This is in contrast to the presently used forms of treatment, which clumsily destroy many normal cells along with the tumor cells, causing much damage. The specificity of monoclonal antibodies has the potential for avoiding unnecessary suffering.

A drawback to the use of monoclonals in human cancer is neutralization by the body. Monoclonals are made from stimulated B cells of animals that have been injected with the human tumor. Antibodies may be formed in the patient against the foreign immunoglobulins, thus inactivating them. As technology improves, monoclonals will probably be made from human cells, to make them more compatible with the body.

In spite of the many problems that still have to be solved, the potential of monoclonals in cancer therapy is exhilarating. Some positive preliminary results have been reported in patients with certain leukemias, gastrointestinal cancer, and lymphomas. Custom-made monoclonals were able to achieve remissions! Antibodies can be used as tools, limited only by our imagination.

Monoclonals can also be used as a passive form of immunotherapy in immunosuppressed individuals who don't make their own antibodies. The immunosuppression may be temporary, perhaps due to toxic drugs or radiation exposure. After the cause is removed, it frequently takes months before the immune system returns to normal. In the meantime, the patient is susceptible to all kinds of infections, even from bugs that ordinarily are not troublesome. Laboratory-made stocks of monoclonal antibodies, against the various common pathogens of the environment, could be administered to save lives during the interim period.

In the battle against diseases, making use of the same natural products that the body normally uses to maintain health makes good sense. Amplifying the immune system can force it to put up a stronger fight. Once all the weapons in nature's immune arsenal are identified, the power to tip the balance in our favor may finally be realized. Reinforcing our natural defenses to control disease could become a prime factor for improving quality of life and longevity.

Summary

Without the meddling of immunologists, life on earth would be a constant struggle to remain alive. Many dread diseases have been conquered by cleverly manipulating the resources we were endowed with. Several aspects of the immune system must be escalated in order to secure the upper hand in the competition between man and his predators.

The economic progress of the world is also intricately tied to the accomplishments of immunologists. Loss of productivity due to frequent epidemics and the cost of medical care are usually estimated in the millions of dollars. Manipulation of the immune system has already proved its worth over a long period of time.

Vaccination was one of the earliest techniques developed to enable us to outdo the pathogens. It provides a quick strike against invaders. Vaccines are prepared from attenuated organisms. They cajole the immune system into making a response, as if they were the real thing. The experience comes in handy whenever an encounter with similar organisms occurs. Then the immune apparatus is prepared to strike quickly without any delay. The transgressors are promptly neutralized and cannot establish a foothold. It is the aim of the immunologist to wise up the immune system by exposing it to the likeness of all who prey on us. Vaccines are the ultimate dream for the conquest of many diseases, ranging from the common cold to cancer and AIDS.

We have other biological tricks and agents which can augment the immune apparatus. These aids are part of the system's own repertoire. They include interferon, interleukin-2, tumor necrosis factor, colony-stimulating factors, thymosin, monoclonal antibodies, and many others, even some not yet identified. Each is a link which plays a unique role in our natural defense system. When used alone, the results are frequently frustrating. However, after each has been studied individually, the plan is to put them back together again, to enhance the body's own defenses more effectively.

Since the magnitude of the competition between man and the microbes is great, and the struggle unrelenting, we have been able to target only a few of our opponents so far. For those diseases that still need to be addressed, we can only rely on the intricate workings of a healthy immune system. When it fails, there is trouble. Of course, there are antibiotics and other drugs to fight diseases. But, persistent organisms are frequently able to outdo these weapons, by mutating and developing resistance to the drugs. Immune neutralization of pathogens is the ultimate deterrent. When working well, its effectiveness is so great that we take it for granted. It toils unassumingly, constantly alert for the diseases that wait for an opportunity to pounce. No one can live a normal life without an immune system, and immune modulation is the hope for the future.

4

Disorders of the Immune System

The protective function of the immune system is necessary for survival. Children who are born with major immune deficiencies are defenseless and frequently die at an early age. There is no other bodily mechanism that can cope with the ever-present pathogens that invade from the environment. Likewise, the immune system must be on guard constantly to cope with the scourge from within, when cells change to become tumor cells. Without immune defenses, cancer would reign free.

Occasionally, the benefactor becomes cantankerous. It uses its destructive weapons that normally rid the body of disease to function against the body that nurtures it. Respect for self tissue can be lost. Some body parts are recognized as antigens and are treated like foreign intruders. The result is tissue damage known as autoimmune disease. The term "horror autotoxicus" was coined in 1900 for such conditions.

It is ironic that a system which was designed to protect can also harm. When good, it is very, very good, but when bad, it can be detrimental to the well-being of the body.

AUTOIMMUNE DISEASES

During the early development of the immune system, as far back as fetal beginnings, it learns to tolerate self components. The tolerance is usually maintained until the system begins to decline in old age. Then, autoantibodies against normal tissues sometimes appear. Coincidentally, there may be a decrease in the number of suppressor T cells, so the immune reaction is not held back. The lack of T_s restraint is one of the factors that can allow clones of anti-self lymphocytes to sprout and produce autoantibodies.

Immune damage to self tissues can also develop in younger individuals. Autoantibodies have been found after physical trauma to an organ or infection. If the damage exposes internal components, which have always been hidden from the immune system, they may be mistaken as foreign. The immune cells have not been educated to tolerate sequestered, self antigens. Then, when inappropriately exposed, there may be a rejection reaction.

Some diseases of the thyroid gland are due to autoantibodies which are made against proteins that are normally locked inside the gland. The proteins become exposed to the immune system when the gland is damaged by an infectious agent, or it is physically injured. Complement is attracted and the process of destruction ensues.

Some cases of male infertility may be due to autoantibodies against sperm. Sperm may enter the blood supply during a physical injury, or due to blocked ducts, or disease. They become exposed to circulating lymphocytes which have never been educated to tolerate sperm. Under normal conditions, sperm are hidden from the immune system, since they are shed to the outside. An inadvertent exposure stimulates an anti-sperm response to the "foreign" antigen. The newly formed antibodies enter the seminal fluid and complex with the sperm, thereby preventing motility. The annihilation process is initiated and impaired fertility results.

Self attack may also occur if a virus becomes attached to a cell, and alters its appearance. The combination of cell and virus is recognized as foreign, and the whole complex is destroyed by immune cells.

A viral infection and an autoimmune response are suspected triggers for multiple sclerosis (MS). However, the exact cause still remains shrouded in mystery, since no specific MS virus has been isolated. Genetic factors, which may determine the severity of the disease, are also suspected. The sheath that surrounds nerve cells is attacked by autoreactive lymphocytes. The destruction results in denuded nerves that malfunction. Muscular weakness, visual problems, and slurred speech result, and the disease may progress to paralysis. The lesions contain all the telltale ingredients of an immunologic response, including plasma cells, lymphocytes, and IgG. Frequently the patient has a selective decrease in T_s cells which are needed to counteract the attack on the nerve sheaths.

MS is devastating to young adults. It is the most common degenerative neurological disease that strikes at the height of life, frequently becoming progressive and crippling. There are drugs that lessen the symptoms, but they don't alter the course of the disease. A cure remains elusive, since it awaits unraveling more of the mysteries about the complex immune system.

A drug reaction is suspected in some autoimmune blood cell diseases. If the drug inadvertently binds to the surface membrane of a blood cell, and stimulates the production of antidrug antibodies, the innocent cell becomes a victim of the attack against the drug. When complement is fixed, the whole complex is lysed. The cells are caught in the crossfire. If the cells involved are red cells, their destruction causes anemia. If the drug is absorbed on to platelets, clotting is obstructed, and there is excessive bleeding. When attached to PMN leukocytes, defense against infection is impaired. Fortunately, when the drug is stopped, the destructive immune response is usually terminated. Ironically, the immune reaction is normal in this autoimmune disease, but it is not precisely contained.

An autoimmune reaction can also result from the introduction of a foreign antigen into the body, which resembles a normal tissue antigen. The alien antigen may be different enough to be recognized as foreign by immune cells, but the antibodies that develop cross-react and operate against the normal tissue also. It is called molecular mimicry. Both the foreign antigen and the normal tissue are destroyed by the immune response.

An example is nerve damage, which frequently occurs in patients with a small cell lung cancer, also called "oat cell" cancer. The cancer cells produce neuroendocrine secretions, which are almost similar to those from neural tissues. A lymphocyte response is made against the tumor, but the immune products also recognize normal neural tissues. An autoimmune reaction develops, resulting in nerve impairment and brain degeneration.

A similar autoimmune reaction is believed to be responsible for the development of rheumatic fever, which involves destruction of heart tissue. Autoantibodies that operate against the heart are present in patients infected with certain strains of streptococcus bacteria. The immune system makes antibodies to fight the bacterial infection, but coincidentally they cross-react with innocent heart tissue. Some of the determinants on both are similar. Rheumatic fever usually shows up about 2 weeks after a sore throat that is caused by the offending strain of streptococcus. The timing coincides with the time that it takes to produce the anti-streptococci antibodies. Heart tissue is destroyed when the antibody is deposited on the heart cells, and complement becomes fixed. The whole complex is lysed. Strep throat infections must be treated with antibiotics immediately to prevent crippling complications.

In rheumatoid arthritis (RA), parts of the immune mechanism go awry. Autoantibodies are formed that are known as rheumatoid factor (RF). They unite with the individual's own IgG antibodies. The IgG antibody becomes the antigen for the RF autoantibody. The complex settles in the joints. Complement is attracted, which summons scavenger macrophages and PMN leukocytes to the area. The complexes are frequently too large for some of the phagocytes to engulf. Instead, their destructive enzymes and toxic oxygen products are spilled sloppily to the outside to digest away the complex. Innocent bystander tissue is caught in the middle of the turmoil and eroded away. Disfigurement results. The complement also stimulates local mast cells and basophils to release histamine. Histamine causes blood vessels in the joint to dilate and become permeable, which results in swelling, pain, and redness.

Rheumatoid arthritis is a common disease which is responsible for crippling millions of people. More females are affected than males. Sometimes spontaneous remissions occur, especially during pregnancy; but afterwards it usually worsens again. What triggers the RF formation against the IgG is unknown. Likewise, there is little information to explain the lack of normal suppression by T_s cells. Genetic factors for susceptibility to an undetermined environmental factor may be involved.

Systemic lupus erythematosus (SLE) is an immune complex disease that results from a derangement in the control of normal tolerance to self. Various antibodies are formed against the diverse components of normal body cells. They unite to form complexes of different sizes, which circulate throughout the body, and can settle in many different organs. The complexes attract complement and phagocytes, which ultimately destroy bystander tissues.

When the deposits settle in the joints, arthritis results. Kidney involvement can result in renal disease. Deposits in blood vessels of the skin cause a rash. In some patients, a red, angry-looking rash appears across the nose and cheeks, which resembles a butterfly or wolf's head. The name, lupus erythematosus, means red wolf. The disease may be localized or systemic, involving many organ systems. For each individual disease, a differential diagnosis must be made to determine if SLE is involved.

SLE is most common in young women. The cause is not well understood, but it is evident that many cases follow sensitization by drugs or viruses. A genetic tendency is suspected. A deficiency of suppressor T cells may be involved, which are needed to counteract the inappropriate attack. The condition is exacerbated by oral contraceptives that contain estrogen.

Glomerulonephritis frequently occurs in children who have recently come down with a strep throat. The culprit is a toxin, produced by a certain strain of streptococcus. It is a small molecule which stimulates the production of an antibody. The complex of antigen and antibody is also small, so it circulates readily in the blood vessels. Eventually, it becomes trapped by the kidneys, which are filtering organs. Complement is attracted and the cycle of destruction of bystander, innocent kidney tissue commences.

The manifestations of the disease can be terrifying to the young patient and the parents. An early sign is blood in the urine. The color can range from dark reddish brown to red to smoky. The volume is usually reduced due to kidney damage. Puffiness of facial features and legs results. Happily, a large percentage of patients recover completely with time. Prevention involves early diagnosis of a strep throat, so antibiotics may be started immediately.

Other small antigens, such as circulating drugs or pathogens, can also initiate immune complex glomerulonephritis. The self hurt is always due to the body's own nonspecific assailants, which are attracted to the trapped complexes. When the antigen disappears, the destruction stops.

There is another form of glomerulonephritis, which is due to antigens associated with kidney tissue itself. Changes occur in the kidneys that make them appear foreign and antigenic. The usual perpetrators are viral infections, drugs, or physical damage to the kidneys, which alter their familiar appearance. The modified kidney tissue is recognized as alien and antibodies are produced. The complexes are part of the kidney structure, rather than settled complexes that originated elsewhere.

A form of diabetes, known as type I, insulin-dependent, has autoimmune manifestations. Autoantibodies are present in the serum which react with pancreatic cells that normally produce insulin. The IgG - pancreatic cell complex attracts the nonspecific components of the immune system and a breakdown commences. Insulin can no longer be produced.

Autoimmune diseases are treated with drugs that lessen the angry immune reaction by suppressing the immune system. They don't cure or eliminate the underlying causes, but they lessen the number of immune cells that can cause trouble. The search for better therapies continues.

There are some autoimmune responses that serve useful purposes. They do the work of a sanitation department, to clear away worn-out body cells. The has-beens are recognized as foreign and eliminated. The antibody reaction can also regulate normal immune responses. Production of antibodies must be stopped after they have incapacitated all of their antigens. Antiantibodies are formed to neutralize them. New antibodies recognize the oldies that are no longer needed, and treat them as antigens. It is a feedback system to prevent antibodies from functioning unnecessarily. The network of checks and balances supplements the work of suppressor T cells, which also suppress immune reactions.

HYPERSENSITIVITIES—ALLERGIC DISEASES

Hyperactive immune responses to certain antigens can cause tissue damage. Susceptible individuals have an exaggerated reaction to some foreign agents, like pollen or house dust, that are innocuous and not harmful in themselves. The result is hypersensitivity or allergic disease. It occurs in approximately 10 percent of the population. Four different components of the immune system have been identified that can produce hypersensitivities. Each involves a different aspect of the immune response. Some are antibody-mediated, while others involve CMI. They are classified as Types I–IV.

Type I—Immediate Hypersensitivity (IH)

Inhaling a pollen grain is handled competently and uneventfully by the nonallergic individual. Specific IgG antibodies are made against the pollen. An antigen-antibody complex is formed, and the whole thing is removed by the nonspecific assistants, including complement and phagocytes. There are no unpleasant events.

On the other hand, in allergic individuals, IgE antibody is produced against the pollen grain, rather than IgG. The IgE binds to the local mast cells in the tissues and to basophils in the blood, causing these cells to release their granules when the antigen becomes bound (Figure 4–1). The contents of the granules are highly reactive, especially the histamine component. In a matter of minutes, there is tissue swelling, redness, and leakage of fluids from the blood. It is an immediate hypersensitivity

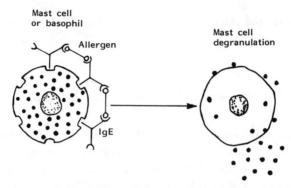

Figure 4–1. **Type I immediate hypersensitivity reaction. Allergens combine with specific IgE antibodies which became attached to the surface of basophils and mast cells. Binding stimulates degranulation and release of chemical mediators.**

reaction (IH). The symptoms vary, depending on the area of the body affected. If the mast cells in the nose are activated, the result is sneezing, and an itchy, runny nose which is red, swollen, and obstructed. The eyes may become involved, with redness and tears; the ears feel full. An allergen which is ingested stimulates IgE, which degranulates mast cells in the gastrointestinal tract. Vomiting and diarrhea may result. Hives may develop in the skin. The consequences of released mast cell granules in the lungs are constricted airways, swelling of the membranes, and obstructions with mucus and fluids. It becomes difficult for air to get through, so there is wheezing and gasping for breath. The condition may evolve into life-threatening asthma. Although the perpetrators are minor, innocuous antigens, the consequences for a susceptible individual are major. Some common allergens include pollens, feathers, animal dander, bacterial products, insect debris, dust, or even ordinary cold air.

A generalized reaction can result when mast cells and basophils are activated throughout the body all at once. This occurs if the antigen is introduced into the bloodstream of a susceptible person by means of an injection or an insect sting. It is circulated rapidly to all parts. As the mast cells degranulate everywhere, huge amounts of histamine are released. The blood vessels become permeable, causing a seepage of fluids from the circulation into the tissues. The extensive fluid loss causes a drop in blood pressure; ultimately it may lead to shock. Respiratory failure can result from severe bronchial spasms, which prevent intake of air. This hypersensitivity reaction is called anaphylaxis. Immediate treatment is crucial to stop the histamine release, and to restore the circulating fluid volume. Otherwise, death comes on rapidly.

A bee sting can cause a generalized reaction in a sensitized individual, since venom is injected into the circulation. When the specific IgE that recognizes the venom is already locked onto the mast cells from a previous experience, the histamine release is rapid. The condition becomes life-threatening. Individuals who know they are sensitive to insect venom may be advised to carry an emergency kit to control the reaction, in case of a future sting.

An injection of penicillin can also produce a generalized response in a penicillin-sensitized individual. As the antigen reaches all areas of the body, a shock reaction can develop. There may be itchy, burning hives, and rashes covering the entire body. Swelling of the larynx may be experienced, which can close off the air passages. It can be fatal if not suppressed immediately. A record of individual drug sensitivities should be carried by all persons at all times. If there is an accident, with loss of consciousness, the instructions carried in a wallet could prevent a life-threatening emergency.

Treatments are available that minimize allergic reactions. When the allergen is seasonal, immunotherapy is employed in anticipation of an encounter. The aim of preseasonal regimens is to build up IgG antibodies to the allergen, slowly, over a period of time. Later, whenever the allergen is encountered, it becomes united with the available IgG, before IgE production can be activated. Elimination of the complex with IgG occurs normally.

Immunotherapy can relieve the annoying symptoms in about 80 percent of patients.

Type II—Antibody-Mediated Cytotoxicity

Cell damage may be caused by an antibody that is made against a surface determinant on a cell. An example is the Rh factor, which is present on red blood cells of Rh$^+$ persons. Most individuals have the dominant, or Rh$^+$ characteristic. A small percentage of people are Rh$^-$. A child born to an Rh$^-$ mother and an Rh$^+$ father expresses the dominant Rh$^+$ determinant. Some of the Rh$^+$ cells of the baby are introduced into the mother's circulation, when there is bleeding at the time of birth. An IgG antibody reaction is instigated in the Rh$^-$ mother, against the baby's Rh$^+$ red cells. The first baby is spared, because the reaction doesn't develop in the mother until after its birth. However, the mother's long-lasting IgG antibodies can operate against the Rh$^+$ fetus in a subsequent pregnancy. The IgG diffuses through the placenta and complexes with the Rh$^+$ red blood cells of the second child. Complement is activated and destruction follows. Rh disease can kill the baby.

Immunologists have learned to successfully avoid Rh destruction in the Type II reaction by means of passive immunity. Antibody production in the Rh$^-$ mother is inhibited at the time of the first birth by injecting the mother with preformed antibodies that are active against Rh$^+$ red cells. The injection is given before she has had a chance to make her own antibodies. They complex with all the Rh$^+$ red cells of the baby that managed to get into her blood. Removal by the accessory system ensues, leaving no antigen to actively stimulate her own antibody formation. Conquering Rh disease is one of the major triumphs of immunology.

Another Type II reaction can occur when drugs or chemicals inadvertently adhere to the surface membranes of cells. If the foreign chemical stimulates antibody formation, the innocent cells are eliminated along with the chemical. The symptoms produced depend on the type of cell which is lost.

Type III—Immune Complex Disorders

Type III diseases involve very small foreign antigens that disperse freely in the blood. They unite with the antibody that is formed against them, and the tiny complexes also circulate throughout the body. Eventually they settle out in different areas. Complement is activated, and an inflammatory reaction ensues. Normal tissues that harbor the complexes are destroyed, due to close association with the products of immune cells that were meant for the foreign invader. The diseases produced also come under the category of autoimmune disorders. These have been discussed with glomerulonephritis and SLE.

Reactions of Types II and III are much slower in forming than Type I. Type I, immediate hypersensitivity, depends on IgE and shows up in a few minutes. Types II and III are IgG reactions. They take several hours to develop, because they require the assistance of the complement cascade and activation of accessory cells. Mustering the additional help adds several hours to the formation of the response.

Type IV—Cell-Mediated Hypersensitivity

The only hypersensitivity diseases that are not mediated by antibodies belong to Type IV. Cell-mediated immunity (CMI) is the culprit. It involves the interaction of T_D lymphocytes with certain antigens. Lymphokines are secreted by the lymphocytes, which activate nonspecific accessory cells. The development of the response is slow, requiring 24 to 72 hours to bring all the players into the act. Type IV lesions are heavily infiltrated with macrophages which are attracted by some of the lymphokines.

In sensitized, allergic individuals, the T_D lymphocytes make an exaggerated reaction to certain chemicals that come into contact with the skin, such as dyes, poison ivy, hair sprays, or metals. Tissue damage results from the activities of the accessory immune cells, rather than from the antigen itself. Phagocytes use their enzymes and toxic oxygen products to eliminate the perpetrators. Innocent bystander tissue becomes destroyed by the released secretions. A rash can develop that is red, swollen, and itchy. The condition is known as contact dermatitis. Genetic factors are believed to be involved in susceptibility to chemical allergens.

IMMUNODEFICIENCY DISEASES

The major immunodeficiency diseases are inherited, and frequently show up in infancy. Such children are born with a lowered resistance to infection. Deficiencies can occur in the humoral system, the cell-mediated immune system, or both. Also, the nonspecific components of defense may be affected.

In a severe humoral deficiency, there are no B lymphocytes anywhere in the body, and no immunoglobulins in the blood. The disease is genetically restricted to male babies. Symptoms first appear after the passively acquired IgG antibodies from the mother are depleted. The baby cannot cope with bacterial infections. T-lymphocyte formation is normal, so intracellular viral infections are resisted. Treatment involves antibiotics and injections of preformed immune serum known as gamma globulin. The immune serum is obtained from normal persons who have long-lasting immunoglobulins. The beneficial effect has a short duration, and must be repeated constantly.

A selective deficiency of only one immunoglobulin class can occur. The most common is an IgA deficiency, which is responsible for repeated colds in children. There is no protection in the bodily fluids at the portals of entry to stop incursions from the environment. The condition is believed to be inherited, or it may be acquired after taking certain drugs which are known to cause a selective IgA deficiency. Cell-mediated immunity is usually normal.

Selective IgM or IgG disorders sometimes develop. Such conditions are rarer than IgA deficiencies.

Individuals who lack T lymphocytes are especially prone to infections by viruses, fungi, parasites, and certain bacteria that live and multiply inside of cells. The condition is due to a defect in the development of the thymus gland. Immature cells, which arrive here from the bone marrow, cannot differentiate. There is an associated abnormality in humoral immunity, since T_H cells must cooperate with B cells for most antibody responses. Treatments which have been tried include implantation of fetal thymus tissue, and injections of the thymic hormone, thymosin.

In combined immunodeficiency disease, both systems of immunity are affected. A defect in bone marrow stem cells prevents normal development of B and T cells. The condition has a genetic basis. Victims are susceptible to all sorts of uncontrollable infections, even from relatively harmless organisms that ordinarily do not cause disease. A completely sterile environment is required for survival.

David, the bubble boy, gained notoriety because he lived in a sterile plastic bubble for many years. He suffered from combined immunodeficiency disease, but was kept alive until his teens. He was tutored through the bubble and made contact with his family through the layer of plastic. For recreation, a customized space suit was constructed, which allowed him to move about while remaining in an antiseptic environment. He died after an attempted bone marrow graft. Fetal liver cell grafts are also used to try to establish immune function.

Inherited disorders can occur that involve nonspecific defenders, such as phagocytes and complement. When either of these systems is defective, there is an increased frequency of infection. Phagocytic cells may be present, but their enzymes can be abnormal. They fail to degrade pathogens. Instead, the ingested organisms thrive and continue to multiply inside the phagocytes. A malfunction in the process of phagocytosis is another genetic anomaly.

Patients with complement deficiencies cannot clear out antigen-antibody complexes. An increased susceptibility to infection results, since antibodies alone are not sufficient protection. They can only recognize and immobilize the antigen. Complement is needed for the final destruction. Deficiencies in one or several components of the complement system can occur. They are genetically determined, and are usually present in more than one family member. Treatment for infections depends on antibiotics.

Some deficiencies of the immune system are acquired during a lifetime, rather than inherited. An immune cell may turn cancerous, involving itself mainly in reproduction, at the expense of its normal function. The patient becomes susceptible to infections. In addition, as the cancer cell aggressively reproduces itself, it can inhibit and destroy other cells, causing multiple symptoms.

A viral infection may impair one type of immune cell, so it can no longer contribute to the network of immune interactions. If it happens to be a pivotal cell, like T_H, the whole defense system falls apart. Patients with AIDS suffer from a loss of T_H function.

A drug, taken for an unrelated disease, may inadvertently suppress or destroy some immune cells. Side effects of drugs need to be monitored, because the results of acquired deficiencies can be as damaging as inherited disorders.

An overall immune senescence develops with age. A consequence is increased susceptibility to infections and cancer in the elderly. An age-associated deficit in tolerance to self tissues can occur.

In this age of prevention, maintaining immune competence should become a prominent goal to reduce the incidence of disease. This is especially pertinent since prevention is frequently more effective than treatment.

SUMMARY

Like an overprotective mother, an overprotective immune system can bring harm. Protection may be extended to innocuous antigens, which ordinarily can cause no trouble. In its overzealousness, the defense system summons all of its helpers and accessories into the act. They blindly create their turmoil, often for no good reason. Hypersensitivity or allergy results. The reactions may be immediate, requiring only minutes to develop, or they may be delayed for several hours or days. Each type of reaction is mediated by different cells, or products of the immune system. Some responses may involve the whole body and can cause instant death due to anaphylaxis.

The immune system may also fail because it loses its ability to distinguish self body parts from nonself intruders. Self antigens normally train lymphocytes, early in their development, to stay away, not to react. However, some self components remain hidden from lymphocytes. These are sequestered antigens that don't participate in the education process. Later, if they become exposed by trauma or disease, the uneducated lymphocytes participate in an angry elimination reaction. They respond as they would towards any foreign intruder, which results in devastating damage to the body that may be fatal.

Immune deficiencies may be inherited or acquired. Genetic inadequacies show up at an early age. They may be lethal. Acquired deficiencies can occur at any time, due to an infection, a drug, or cancer. Strange combinations which alter normal tissues can instigate a wipeout. Vital body parts are destroyed by the body's own system of defense.

5

Transplantation

The purpose of a good immune system is to prevent all foreign invaders from gaining a foothold in the body. However, the system is not versatile enough to discriminate in favor of intruders that are beneficial. Although some trespassers may be therapeutic, and desperately needed to maintain life, they must also go. Foreignness is the only criterion the immune system uses, and the good foreigners succumb along with the bad, to a stiff-necked and unyielding mechanism. The immune system is the greatest obstacle to most organ transplants.

When defective organs are replaced with healthy ones, a fight usually ensues. Potentially lifesaving grafts from other persons are rejected, because the transplanted tissues carry genetically determined antigens that are unique to each individual.

These are the foreign culprits that trigger an attack when outside their own milieu. The assault can culminate in rejection. The greater the number of antigenic differences between graft and host, the faster the rejection response. Conversely, the closer the genetic relationship, the greater the probability of a "take." As with any other immune reaction, the lymphocyte clones that develop against the alien tissue have specificity and memory. A second transplant, which bears antigens similar to the first, is rejected faster than the original. Only the organs of identical twins have the same determinants, and can be freely exchanged with impunity.

The cells responsible for rejection are mainly T lymphocytes of the host. Killer T cells (T_K) respond to the foreign tissues in the same way as they react against their own tissues when they become altered by a virus or a tumor antigen. The challenge triggers cell division and clone formation. The army of mature T_K cells makes direct contact with the cells of the graft, and attacks with a lethal hit which damages the graft. T_H and T_D lymphocytes are also present at the rejection site. Lymphokines are secreted that attract macrophages and other accessory cells to the area. Each cell type inflicts its own special injury, which contributes to the destructive process. The combined clobbering culminates in the final rejection of the precious graft.

Foreign grafts also stimulate a humoral response, but antibodies don't appear to play a major role in graft rejection. In fact, there is evidence that they may protect the graft. By forming complexes with antigens on the surface of the graft, they conceal them from the attacking T_K cells. Thus, they become "blocking antibodies" that sometimes help to extend the life of incompatible grafts.

Since it is virtually impossible to find organ donors who have tissue antigens similar to the prospective host, unless they are identical twins, immunosuppressive therapy is required to maintain a graft. The host lymphocytes must be suppressed to minimize their attack on the surgically inserted foreign organ.

The transplant must be shielded from the reacting lymphocytes, for the lifetime of the graft.

Taming the immune system into submission is very costly to the well-being of the patient. The suppressive treatments in use are relatively nonspecific, causing a generalized interference with cell division. Lymphocytes that are not even involved with the graft, and are needed to form clones to block the ever-present pathogens in our environment, are inhibited. The price that must be paid by transplant patients is an increase in the incidence of infectious diseases and cancer. Immune tumor surveillance is mercilessly impaired.

MATCHING

In spite of the problems with rejection, organs which are obtained from live, unrelated donors, and cadavers have been successfully transplanted. Careful matching helps to insure success. Of course, the best results involve exchanges with tissues that bear similar determinants. These can only be obtained from self, as is possible with skin grafts, or from identical twins. There is no immune fight. Unfortunately, the frequency of twinning is only 1 in approximately 250 births. So, the majority of us lack a carbon copy.

Recently, the mother of a teenage boy came to a transplant surgeon's office accompanied by her son. He was on dialysis due to kidney disease, and desperately wanted a new kidney. The mother had firmly made up her mind. She came to offer her kidney, so her son could return to a normal life. "No," the surgeon replied, "I prefer to use a sibling." He went on to explain that when either parent serves as a donor for a child, there has to be at least a 50 percent match and a 50 percent mismatch. The child inherits half his traits from each parent. Some matches between nonidentical siblings offer better odds for success. Sibling genes are handed down from the same set of parents. The match between any pair of siblings may range from almost completely matched, 50 percent matched, or completely mismatched. The greater the mismatch, the speedier the rejection process. The closer the match, the less immunosuppressive therapy required. The damage to the general well-being of the patient is less.

The frustration and disappointment were overwhelming to both mother and son. They hardly spoke to one another on the way home. Instead, they each relived the buildup that led to the decision the boy had first opposed. Now, it collapsed with a simple no. The struggle that presently confronted the mother was incomparably more painful than prevailing on her son to accept her kidney. This time it involved one of her two healthy children. Another child would be put in jeopardy, in addition to her dialysis child.

Close matches with nonrelatives are difficult to obtain. Compatibility or matching tests are always performed to select a donor who may have at least some transplantation antigens in common with the recipient. Also, the blood type must be similar, since the A, B, and O antigens of red blood cells are also present on many other cells of the body. Blood type differences can also cause rejections.

Privilege

Some locations in the body have few blood vessels and the lymphatic drainage is poor. Unrelated grafts made into these areas have a good chance of defying the rejection process, since circulating lymphocytes are sparse. The foreign antigens of such grafts cause minimal sensitization of immune cells of the host. These areas are known as "privileged sites."

A cornea graft to the eye occupies a privileged site, and is usually well tolerated. It is the most common transplantation procedure performed, since the chances for tissue survival are good, even when unrelated donors are used. Each year, sight is successfully restored to thousands of people by giving them new corneas. Eye banks have been organized to harvest and store the tissue, which can be obtained from cadavers. It is a tissue that can await the proper host but, unfortunately, the demand exceeds the supply. Few recipients develop complications, although occasionally some need to be treated for rejection.

Tissues of the brain occupy a favored site, since lymphoid drainage is absent from the central nervous system. Some neurosurgeons feel that the potential for graft survival is good. Destroyed brain parts are being replaced in some victims of Parkinson's disease to restore lost function. If a diseased part can be successfully supplanted, why couldn't we also plan for transplants to enhance brain power? The use of surrogate brain fragments is intriguing, and may someday occupy the attention of scientists.

Some tissues are naturally cooperative grafts, because of their structure. They are "privileged tissues" that are able to survive most of the time, due to built-in barriers which inhibit their interaction with immune cells of the host. Such tissues include tendons with their covering sheaths, ligaments, cartilage, bone, and heart valves. They are well tolerated, and usually escape rejection, even from unmatched donors.

The amount of tissue transplanted also influences tolerance. There is a dose response, since small transplants present fewer antigens than larger tissues. The small size of the cornea graft contributes to its favorable acceptance rate.

The age of the recipient is important in the rejection reaction. When newborns receive transplants, the fight is feeble, because the immune apparatus is immature. Tolerance is good. Also, the number of suppressor T cells is high in the young, which can dampen an angry immune response. The T_s cells contribute to the down-modulation of a potential rejection.

Experiments with infant mice have demonstrated the acceptance of foreign antigenic cells. Throughout life, these cells remain tolerated. The young lymphocytes of the host become educated to the foreign presence, and soon treat it as self tissue. Grafts from the same donor that are made at a later date are usually accepted also. As long as the new tissues bear the same genetically determined antigens as the original transplanted cells, they are tolerated. How convenient it would be if every newborn baby could be paired with a transplant partner. They would be insurance for each other to protect against a failed kidney, or the need for skin that was destroyed in a fire, later in life. Imaginative immunologists can set the stage for much future research.

CONTROL OF REJECTION

The pretransplant matching and compatibility tests help to select donors whose tissues will provoke the least amount of rejection in the recipient. However, there are many transplantation antigens which have not been identified as yet, and tests are not available. Therefore, it is impossible to attain total compatibility, unless the donor and recipient are identical twins. Consequently, most transplant patients are saddled with a lifetime of drugs, which protect their replacement organs from rejection. Lymphocytes that are stimulated by the mismatched antigens must be continuously suppressed. This might be tolerable if the drugs were as specific as the lymphocyte clones that cause the rejection. Evolution has succeeded in developing finely tuned lymphocyte specificities, one for each antigen, but man's attempts at selectivity to counteract only the special clones involved in the rejection reaction have been clumsy, so far. The conventional immunosuppressants in use are mostly generalized killers that stop cell division nonspecifically. A complication of the treatment is widespread damage to lymphoid cells that are needed for protection, and injury to other cells that are actively dividing in the body. Immunosuppressive therapies involve the use of chemical, physical, and biological agents.

Chemical Agents of Suppression

Most of the chemical agents prescribed for transplant patients are similar to those used for chemotherapy against cancer. A weakened immune response results from the treatments, making the patient prey to attack by opportunistic pathogens and cancer.

The advent of the antibiotic, cyclosporine, has improved the prognosis for organ grafts. It is an anti-rejection drug with some selectivity, since it is specific for T_H lymphocytes, the pivotal cell in the immune network (Figure 2-3). With no T_H, the T_H-dependent cells like T_K cannot participate in the rejection response. Graft survival is prolonged. In addition, cyclosporine enhances the activity of suppressor T lymphocytes. T_S cells contribute to a state of graft tolerance by modulating the angry immune attack. Since the inhibitory effect involves only T_H cells, other dividing cells in the body are not affected. Most blood-forming cells of the bone marrow are not suppressed, so the nonspecific elements of the immune system can continue to operate against infectious agents. With cyclosporine therapy, wound healing is not impeded, and the incidence of infectious diseases is less than with the other immunosuppressive drugs.

However, like most drugs, cyclosporine has harmful side effects, too. It is toxic to kidneys and liver, making it necessary to monitor the serum concentration of the drug periodically. When toxicity develops, cyclosporine must be withdrawn. Unfortunately, the favorable effect on the graft is quickly reversed, so other therapies or combinations have to be substituted. In addition, cyclosporine reduces surveillance against newly developing cancer cells, since the pivotal T_H cells are suppressed. All transplantation patients are more susceptible to malignancies than the general population.

Physical Suppression

Physical treatments involve radiation therapy to the lymphoid organs to suppress reactive cells. The toxicity of radiation is nonselective, involving all lymphoid cells that are hit, as well as any other cells in the vicinity. Graft survival is prolonged, but there are risks for infections and cancer. Radiation is used mainly in animal experimentation.

Biological Agents of Suppression

Large doses of corticosteroid hormones are used. They diminish rejection by decreasing the number of lymphocytes in the circulation. Of course, defense against infectious agents and tumors is weakened. In addition, long-term use of high doses of corticosteroids should be avoided because they have side effects which can result in impaired wound healing, gastrointestinal problems, reactivation of tubercular lesions, and osteoporosis.

A biological immunosuppressive agent with some selectivity is antithymocyte serum. Antibodies are made against human T cells by immunizing horses, sheep, goats, or rabbits. The isolated human T cells are injected into the animals which recognize them as foreign. Antibodies against the T cells soon appear in the serum. When antibody fraction is injected into a transplant patient, the reactive immunoglobulins combine selectivity with the human T cells and inactivate them. Lymphocyte activity against the graft is reduced, whereas other body cells in division are not affected. The limitation of the procedure is a hypersensitivity reaction which may develop against the foreign animal serum. Also, other T-cell activities are stymied.

A monoclonal antibody, made from a hybridoma, has been approved by the FDA (Food and Drug Administration) to counteract kidney rejection. It operates against a surface determinant that is present on 95 percent of mature human T cells. Clones of lymphocytes which would naturally form against the graft are squelched. Unfortunately, it is a generalized T-cell suppressant, since it targets a majority of mature T cells. The body becomes deprived of other T-cell functions as well.

KIDNEY TRANSPLANTS

Kidneys are transplanted more frequently than any other organ. In many cases, it is the treatment of choice for a failing kidney, enabling the patient to return to a normal life. The grafts are obtained either from live donors or cadavers. The great success of kidney transplants may be attributed to the availability of organs from matched family members. The donor can live with a single kidney, while the patient has a better chance of holding on to his related graft, than if it came from the population at large. The survival rate for unrelated cadaver kidneys is always less.

When confronted with a kidney rejection that doesn't respond to immunosuppressive therapy, all is not lost. A new kidney can be substituted. Many patients are alive today who have had more than three transplants. Most patients prefer the grafts to other forms of treatment.

BONE MARROW TRANSPLANTS

Bone marrow is the most important source of cells for the blood and immune system. Anything that goes wrong in the marrow can cause severe changes in the body, which may become life-threatening.

The various cell types produced by the bone marrow descend originally from a single stem cell, which gives rise to different lineages. A deficiency in any one of the lines can result in disease. With abnormalities in red cell progenitors, anemia develops. Blood clotting can be altered by anomalies in the source of platelets. Deviant prelymphocytes can cause lymphocytic cancers, and deficiencies of either the humoral system, CMI, or both. The nonspecific phagocytes also originate in the bone marrow, and can suffer defects due to aberrations here. Bone marrow may be considered the wellspring of life.

Abnormalities that occur in the marrow may necessitate a transplant. Although the procedure is simple, the problems with bone marrow transplants can be great. The marrow is usually drawn out of the pelvic bones of the donor with a syringe (Figure 1–1). It is then prepared for infusion into a vein of the recipient, like an ordinary blood transfusion. The donor cells make their way to the recipient's bone marrow and set up shop.

As with all other transplants, compatibility testing must be done to obtain a decent match, and minimize the rejection response. However, the nature of the graft can cause complications. The donor marrow contains competent, mature T lymphocytes, the very same cells that are capable of participating in graft rejection, when they exist in their own body. In their new surroundings, the donated cells continue to react against the foreign antigens on the cells of the host. Ironically, the grafted lymphocytes reject the host in a graft-versus-host reaction (GvH). This condition develops mainly in immature or immunologically suppressed individuals, whose own lymphocytes are not able to keep the grafted cells in check.

Young children who need bone marrow transplants usually do not have competent lymphocytes of their own. The grafted marrow cells enjoy free reign. They form clones that home into the young host's lymphoid organs throughout his body. Here they continue to expand their forces, always stimulated by the foreign antigens they encounter. The donor cells raid and plunder, until they are stopped eventually by the death of the host.

Adults who are immunologically impotent are also susceptible to the GvH disease. It is common in cases of leukemia, where there is a deficiency of competent lymphocytes. With no restraints against them, the replacement marrow cells grab the opportunity to take over, ravaging the host. High levels of radiation also destroy bone marrow cells, so that grafting becomes complicated by GvH disease.

Recently, the chances for survival after bone marrow grafting have been greatly increased by procedures which treat donated marrow cells in the test tube, prior to infusion into the host. One technique utilizes monoclonal antibodies against mature T cells. They are added to the bone marrow mixture, together with complement (C). The mature T cells become attached to the specific antibodies and the complement lyses the complex. The cells are purged from the donor marrow, before they are transplanted. Only young T cells remain in the graft. They are too immature to become activated by the foreign antigens of the new host. Instead, the young cells learn to become tolerant of their surroundings as they continue on with their differentiation. The survival statistics for bone marrow recipients have been dramatically improved by the processed marrow.

Another technique makes use of a binding agent from soybeans to agglutinate the culprit cells. Mature T cells become bound, and they can be separated and removed from the mixture before implantation into the recipient.

With a successful marrow transplant, the grafted cells gradually repopulate the marrow and lymphoid organs of the host. During this time, the patient must be protected from all pathogens, because of extreme vulnerability to infections. He is defenseless while awaiting reconstitution by a new immune mechanism, which can take several months to become fully functional. Eventually, an effective transplant can bring a patient back to full health.

Another procedure, which is sometimes used, involves infusions of liver cells from a fetus. In the early weeks of life, before bone marrow is developed, the forerunners of blood and immune cells appear in the liver. Later in development, these stem cells migrate to the newly formed spaces in the bones which become the marrow. If an aborted fetus is available, its liver is a good source of precious stem cells to repopulate bone marrow. The immaturity of the cells makes them less likely to instigate the deadly GvH disease.

HEART TRANSPLANTS

New hearts are adding years of life to previously doomed individuals. The surgical techniques have been perfected, and the operation may even be called routine. However, taming the immune system into holding on to the grafted heart remains a subject for ongoing research. At the same time that immunity must be weakened to protect the transplant, opportunistic infections must be curbed. Combinations of biological and chemical immunosuppressive agents have already enabled a large number of patients to survive for several years, but there is still room for improvement in the quality of life.

Another problem is the shortage of donors. The need for hearts is great, but the donation rate is small. Many desperate heart patients die each year while waiting for a new organ. This has led researchers to experiment with interim hearts, to make the waiting period safer. A current research plan involves taking some of the workload off an ailing heart by anastomosing it to a healthy heart, obtained from a chimpanzee. Chimps have been selected since they are closely related to man and have similar blood types. Of course, crossing species barriers is still a source of great aggravation to the immune system. However, the short-term nature of the implant is a factor in overcoming the obstacles. Immunosuppressive agents should control the rejection for the transition period.

PANCREAS TRANSPLANTS

Some diabetic patients are being helped with pancreatic transplants. Candidates for the procedure usually suffer severe complications from their disease, despite insulin therapy. The whole organ may be transplanted or just the insulin-producing cells. When a small amount of tissue is grafted, a living related donor can be used. Immunosuppression is the limiting factor that determines the success rate of these grafts.

OTHER TRANSPLANTS

Immunosuppressive techniques have made possible the replacement of many other types of organs. People have been restored to relatively normal, productive lives with new livers, spleens, and lungs.

Experiments are being conducted to replace destroyed brain parts. Adrenal to brain transplants, which involve tissues from the same individual, are being used to alleviate Parkinson's disease. Also, brain fragments from aborted fetuses have been implanted into the brains of adults who are afflicted with Parkinson's disease. The procedures are experimental and require further testing.

With all transplants, the surgical techniques present few difficulties. The big hurdle is always immune rejection. The goal for the future is the development of more specific suppressants, that function only against those lymphocyte clones that are stimulated by each graft. Perhaps tailor-made monoclonal antibodies will be prepared for each transplant recipient. The effect on longevity statistics could be staggering.

Mechanical Replacement Parts

Another direction for organ transplants involves artificial parts. The immunologic barriers could be bypassed. With the simple mechanics of organs like the heart, this is more of a possibility than with other complicated structures. The heart functions as a pump, which can be replaced by an artificial, man-made pump. Several models are in clinical use, although the quality of life they afford is not always acceptable. So far, the risk of damaged blood cells, clots, and infections have not been overcome. It is best to use these devices as temporary bridges, while waiting for a human heart. Most other organs are so intricately organized that bioengineered replacements still remain in the realm of science fiction.

Summary

The idea of organ transplantation is not new. Since ancient times, medical people have been trying to replace worn-out or deformed parts with new ones that were obtained from unrelated individuals. The grafts never lasted. The immune system is the major impediment to such grandiose ideas.

The barriers to successful transplantation therapy are the genetically determined differences between people. When an organ from an unrelated donor is transplanted, it is recognized as a foreign invader and promptly rejected, like a lowly virus or fungus. We need the immune system for protection, but it needs to be fooled into accepting beneficial intrusions. The possibility of cajoling it into compromising itself, in order to discriminate in favor of grafts, has been occupying scientists for decades. The tinkering has proved to be productive, but the price that has to be paid is high. Purposeful suppression of immune cells allows the grafts to take hold. There can be no rejection without the meddling of lymphocytes. However, most immunosuppressants counteract many different clones of immune cells, leaving the patient defenseless to all the demons in the environment. The treatment must be juggled to obtain a balance between suppression and protection.

It is the aim of immunologists to develop more discerning suppressants. It is hoped that they will wipe out only those clones of lymphocytes that respond specifically to the graft. Evolution has provided us with a system of specificity, in which each lymphocyte is genetically programmed to recognize a different antigen. It is estimated that there are over a million different recognizable specificities. Someday we may be able to match the powers of nature with specific antibodies to stop only those special lymphocytes that operate against each graft. Once we learn how to narrow the opposition, the glitches could be removed from organ transplantation.

6

Tumor Immunology

Theoretically, immunological therapies for cancer make good sense, because fighting cancer is the business of the immune system. There is evidence that immune cells keep a constant vigil in the body, to detect the early emergence of abnormal cells. As soon as the quarry is spotted, an effort is made to annihilate it. However, tumor cells sometimes sneak through the lines and stealthily escape immune surveillance. Once they increase their numbers, an enhanced immune capacity is needed to nab the fugitives more effectively. Cancer immunotherapy attempts to boost the immune system to magnify the body's own response against the disease.

So far, the immunotherapy that is available has not drastically modified the prognosis for cancer. Nevertheless, the use of immunostimulants in different combinations is still believed to be a sensible approach for purging the body of aberrant cells. Many scientists have pinned their hopes on immunotherapy for cancer. Gradually, it is yielding some encouragement.

Some human cancers are resistant to the traditional treatments, which include surgery, radiation, and chemotherapy. Moreover, the latter two regimens are nonspecific inhibitors of all dividing cells of the body, cancerous as well as normal. When there is no specificity, some well-behaved cells that are involved in their proper functions are killed, along with the tumor cells. The results include hair loss, because of the destruction of the rapidly dividing cells of the hair follicles; diarrhea, vomiting, and miserable nausea are the consequences of damage to the normal, constantly renewing epithelial lining of the gastrointestinal tract. Impairment of vital cells of the bone marrow causes anemia, interferes with blood clotting, and destroys desperately needed immune function. Immune cells are prevented from dividing, so specific clones that operate against foreign agents cannot be formed. Paradoxically, these treatments prevent the immune system from participating in the battle against the very cancer cells that are being fought. Virtually all chemotherapeutic drugs and radiation suppress the immune system. The suppression may also be an instigator for future cancer development, since there is a loss of surveillance to counteract the emergence of new cancer cells.

In spite of the recognized drawbacks of chemotherapy and radiation, they are the only accepted treatments we have at the present time. On the positive side, they have resulted in many successful remissions and even cures. Of course, when a remission is effected, the distressful side effects become minor in comparison. It is important to know what to expect with the conventional regimens, and it is always less frightening when you understand why.

An example of the distressing side effects of chemotherapy

is the case of P. F., who was treated for lymphoma. Struggling with the usual nausea and hair loss was hard enough. Fortunately, these were reversible in a short time. But he was not prepared for the more permanent repercussions that followed. As treatment with the prescribed regimen of drugs was nearing completion, he began to develop pain in his legs and feet. It got progressively worse, until his whole body was wracked with frequent attacks of pain. A return visit to the oncologist yielded good news and bad. Happily, no trace of the cancer remained. The chemotherapy had routed that. But there were new problems created by the treatments. He learned that one of the drugs that had to be used may bring on neuritic pain, and later, motor difficulties can follow. Soon it was hard to walk; he couldn't sit for any length of time; he couldn't sleep; he couldn't think. The misery was only slightly relieved by soaking in hot tubs. How could he possibly enjoy life with merciless, unyielding pain? He refused to believe that these neuromuscular deficits could not be reversed. So, he began a trek from the office of one health care specialist to the next, always hoping to find the elusive "Holy Grail." It cost him many months in time, and many, many dollars to arrive at the disappointing realization that he had no choice except to accept the pain. For P. F., pain is part of being alive. It is as commonplace as eating and breathing. The only way to ignore it is by being completely involved in engrossing activities. When his attention is occupied, the pain goes out of focus, and living becomes enjoyable. As a result, he has created a fuller life for himself. His time has become crammed with interesting pursuits, and the pain has been relegated to the background.

The alternate concept for cancer therapy involves enhancement of immune potential, so it can take a more active role in wiping out cancer cells. Both the nonspecific first-line defenders and the specific defense system are enlisted. However, most forms of immunotherapy are still in the experimental stage.

Nonspecific Defenders

Newly transformed cells are first recognized by nonspecific accessory cells of the immune system. The generalists act immediately to destroy many different kinds of emerging tumor cells. There is no need for prior sensitization or clone formation. The natural killer (NK) cells are believed to play an important role in immunity to cancer as well as to viral infections. The macrophages also kill cancer cells nonspecifically, but they must be activated to become killer macrophages.

It is possible that the number of NK cells that are present in an individual at a particular time can influence tumor risk. Unfortunately, NK activity declines with age. Coincidentally, tumors are more prevalent in the aged.

Specific Defenders

Telltale markers on the surface of tumor cells are recognized by lymphocytes of cell-mediated immunity (CMI). However, they require more time to become involved in the fight than the generalists. These specific defenders need to form clones. Each clone operates only against a specific tumor.

The surface markers that stimulate clone formation are known as tumor-associated antigens (TAAs). They are unique to tumor cells, and are not found on normal cells. They attract attention as foreign antigens. The TAAs may be associated with the transformation to malignancy. The cell surface normally controls the uptake and release of substances from the cell. Modifications in the membrane may be needed to adapt to different requirements for raw materials that accompany the chemical processes of abnormal growth. Also, the surface is involved in normal cell-to-cell adhesiveness. In tumor cells, these attachments are weakened, allowing the cells to metastasize or spread.

They aggressively invade normal tissues, and seed many organs. The newly developed tumor TAAs of aberrant cells may be associated with all the facets of change. Fortunately, they become the target of immune cells which specialize in weeding out the numerous cancer cells that are believed to arise during a lifetime.

The T_K lymphocyte of CMI is involved in surveillance against tumor cells. Each T_K is specific for a different TAA. When it detects a change in a normal cell, it is provoked to form a clone. T_H is also involved, since it stimulates T_K formation (Figure 2–3).

In cases where the tumor cells are not rejected, but go on to overwhelm the host, it is believed that inadequate responses were made. The host may not have been immunocompetent during the time of cellular change to malignancy. The fast-growing tumor cells escape surveillance, and the cancer increases to a critical mass. The tumor cells grow out of range for control by the immune system. Immunotherapy aims to support the immune apparatus in its race for supremacy against the cancer.

ESCAPE FROM IMMUNE SURVEILLANCE

There are many explanations to account for the ability of tumor cells to outsmart normal immunologic surveillance. (1) A spontaneous tumor may be weakly antigenic, due to the similarity of its TAAs with conventional self antigens. Cunningly, the tumor tricks the immune cells into ignoring it, and continues to grow unimpeded. (2) The TAAs may not appear early enough on the membranes of the developing clone to alert the immune sentries. A rejection can only occur before the cancer grows large enough to gain the upper hand. Alternatively, the TAAs may appear early, but they occur sparsely on the cell. Their minimal presence cannot be sensed by the lymphocytes. (3) The shedding of fragments from the surface membrane of tumor cells has been

observed with the electron microscope. A TAA on a shed frag-
ment can combine with a cancer-fighting lymphocyte, thus tying
it up and preventing it from functioning against the intact tumor
cell. In the meantime, the cell regenerates new TAAs on its
surface. Free TAAs may also become dispersed as a result of the
destruction of a tumor cell. The immune fighters are wasted on
these segments that can no longer do any harm, anyhow. The
isolated TAA fragments may be compared to the decoys used in
warfare. They are launched to usurp the enemy's defenses, thus
clearing the way for the real offensive weapons. (4) After an
intense host reaction to the specific TAAs on the tumor cells,
mutants or variants of the TAAs may emerge. The mutated TAAs
are able to evade the immune response that was already mustered. Since it takes a long time to develop a new defense, the
fruitful cancer cells make good use of the opportunity to increase
their numbers, to gain the upper hand. (5) Antibodies from the
humoral immune system may be made against the TAAs. Their
effectiveness is diminished when the TAAs are sparse, and
spaced far apart on the membrane. Complement is not attracted
to the complex, so there is no destruction. These tumor antibodies can serve to inhibit a successful CMI response. They cover
up the TAAs like Band-Aids, so they are no longer visible to
killer lymphocytes. Such antibodies are called "blocking antibodies." Inappropriately, they enhance tumor growth. (6) Suppressor T lymphocytes (T_s) have been found in abnormally large
numbers in animals with growing tumors. Normally, they are
part of the network that curtails immune responses, both humoral and CMI, when the reactions have proceeded far enough.
T_s cells in tumorous animals are specific for the TAAs, and they
block an effective immune response. They enable the tumor cells
to escape surveillance. (7) There are some tumor determinants
which are known to preferentially activate T_s cells, rather than
T_K. The suppressors interfere with the activities of the cells involved in the rejection process (Figure 2–3). The host can become tolerant of his own tumor. (8) Some tumor cells produce

mucin, which blankets the surface of the cell and conceals its telltale determinants. The killer cells are prevented from adhering to the TAAs, and cannot inflict the "kiss of death." (9) Genetic determinants, which are part of the individual's heritage, and control the magnitude of his response to the specific tumor antigens, may not favor a strong reaction. The patient is incapable of responding adequately, and becomes tolerant of his tumor.

All of these obstacles must be addressed by the cancer scientist. Each interferes with immune surveillance and may operate to a different degree in different individuals who succumb to cancer. The nature of the tumor, and the condition of the host, influence the prognosis for this dread disease.

CATEGORIES OF TUMOR-ASSOCIATED ANTIGENS (TAAs)

Three major categories of TAAs have been recognized. One is triggered by cancer-causing chemicals, known as carcinogens. Each chemically induced tumor develops its own unique determinants which are distinct from those of other tumors that are spurred by the same carcinogen. Two tumors may even be induced in different areas of the same animal, using the same chemical, and each tumor bears its own special TAAs. This is because there is a random interaction of the chemical with each of the tissues. Each time it is administered, the chemical activates different genes in the cell, the units of heredity, possibly causing different mutations. The altered genes code for different TAAs on the tumor cell surface.

In contrast, the surface determinants of tumors that are induced by viruses are constant. Similar TAAs are present on all the tumors that are induced by the same virus, even in different parts of the body, or in unrelated animal species. The TAA may be part of the viral structure, or it may be an antigen that is induced by the virus. It is a nonvariable determinant.

Some tumor cells have embryonic markers on their surface membranes, which are similar to structures present during early development. They are normal to the fetus in the first few months of life, but later become suppressed, possibly because they are no longer needed. They may be identified on normal fetal yolk sac, liver, and intestine. As the organs mature, they can be found only in trace amounts. A reexpression may occur in cells that are altered by the malignant state. As the cells shift to a pathway of speedy growth, as is characteristic of the fetus, the determinants may become useful once again. It is thought that the genes which code for the expression of fetal determinants are maintained in a suppressed state in the normal adult. They may become reexpressed and code for TAAs in cells that are undergoing malignancy. Two examples of fetal antigens that are associated with human tumors are carcinoembryonic antigen (CEA) and alpha-fetoprotein (AFP). They serve as antigens that are recognized by specific antibodies.

The concentration of CEA in the serum of many patients with colon or pancreatic cancer is especially high. However, it may also be associated with some other forms of cancer. The antigen is shed into the blood, and can be used in a test to determine the status of the tumor. CEA disappears if the tumor regresses, or is surgically removed. It reappears if the tumor recurs. An antibody test for CEA is used to monitor the effects of therapy. Unfortunately, it cannot be used to screen the general population for gastrointestinal cancer, because it can also be found in several noncancerous conditions. CEAs may develop in people with nonmalignant colitis, heavy smokers, and in alcoholics. Perhaps they serve as a forewarning about bad habits.

Alpha-fetoprotein is another determinant that is secreted by some tumor cells, but is also present in the fetus. It is produced normally in the yolk sac and developing liver. Then, it gradually declines. In later years, it may be made by adult tumor tissue, especially by liver cancer cells and other gastrointestinal tumors. Like CEA, it is only used as an indicator, to determine the status of a tumor. After successful therapy, the concentration of AFP declines. If the telltale markers show up again, it indicates a recurrence of the cancer. AFP cannot be used as a general screening test for cancer, because elevated serum levels may also occur in patients with alcoholic liver disease and hepatitis, which would confuse the results.

LINKS TO CANCER

The factors leading to a particular cancer are difficult to assess. This is because many years may elapse from the time of alteration of the single cell to the final diagnosis of cancer. In spite of this, some definite links have already been defined, such as the association of smoking and lung cancer.

A genetic predisposition for a cancer may be present. This does not mean that cancer is directly inherited, but the susceptibility or resistance to agents that can cause the cancer may be inherited. Cancers are more numerous in some families than in others.

Environmental influences may be involved in the alteration of normal cells to cancer cells. They may come from the external or internal milieu. In the outside environment, radiation is a proven physical carcinogen. Numerous chemical pollutants from the environment can also cause changes in susceptible cells. Internal carcinogens may take the form of invading viruses, hormonal imbalances, or chronic irritations.

Poor nutrition has been implicated in promoting cancer. Both excessive eating, which causes overweight, and malnutrition have been correlated with high cancer incidence. The American Cancer Society is promoting a low-fat, low-refined sugar diet, with emphasis on fiber, and elimination of certain food additives that may act as mutagens or carcinogens. It is wise to take preventive measures, whenever risks are suspected, to avert later grief.

EXPERIMENTAL IMMUNOTHERAPIES FOR CANCER

Since many tumor cells have recognizable determinants that are immunogenic, it seems plausible that we should be able to amplify the natural immune response to aid in eliminating the tumor. The treatments that are being explored take advantage of both the nonspecific and specific responses of the immune system. Many of the strategies are being tried experimentally in animals and humans. There are few recognized clinical applications.

BCG

Bacillus Calmette-Guérin (BCG) is a bacterium which causes tuberculosis in cattle. When an attenuated strain is injected into humans, it mobilizes the body's immune resources to function at peak levels. It elevates the activities of T_D and natural killer (NK) cells to initiate attacks against the foreign antigen. At the same time, the aroused defenders and their emissaries also become more lethal to tumor cells that happen to be in the vicinity of the BCG injection. The provoked T_D cells secrete lymphokines, which recruit macrophages to the site. The macrophages are goaded into becoming "killer macrophages." They experience a respiratory burst, puff up, and develop into large, formidable assailants. For speedier action, their motility is increased. They become more sticky, for better holding power; the enemy can't escape. When the victim is ingested, it is subjected to powerful enzymes that degrade it. The lymphokines turn the macrophages into superior killers. They function nonspecifically to rid the site of all foreign antigens, including the tumor cells that are present. The state of activation lasts for several weeks.

The powers of BCG are being utilized for the experimental treatment of some forms of cancer. The "killer macrophages" and NK cells that are aroused need close contact with the tumor cells, at the site of the BCG injection. Therefore, the treatment is most effective when the BCG is injected directly into the lesion. This is possible with accessible tumors, like those in the skin. Some patients with melanoma, a pigment cell cancer, have experienced regressions in a few weeks after being injected with BCG. The successes are limited, however, to accessible nodules. It is also reported to be effective in bladder cancer.

BCG is a promising nonspecific immune treatment. It magnifies some of the body's armamentarium to become more effective in the battle against localized forms of cancer. It will have to be used, together with other treatments, to heighten the entire complex of immune responses, the specific and nonspecific. Immunotherapy for cancer may necessitate a multiple approach.

Removal of Bone Marrow

An immunological technique which attempts to circumvent some of the toxic effects of treatments with radiation and chemotherapy, is bone marrow removal. The precious bone marrow, which is critical for life, contains the stem cells of the blood and immune system. They are most readily destroyed by the high-powered conventional therapies.

To avoid the destruction, the bone marrow may be removed prior to the treatments, to protect it during the onslaught. It is evacuated with a syringe from the pelvic bones or chest bone, and frozen for later reinsertion. In the meantime, the patient is bombarded with toxic doses of chemotherapeutic drugs and radiation to kill all dividing cells. Finally, the thawed marrow is replaced via an intravenous injection. The cells leave the circulation, to home into the marrow and repopulate it.

Complications can affect the success rate of the procedure. Life-threatening infections may occur before the bone marrow becomes reestablished, since it needs several months to regain function. In the meantime, immune potential is low. The normal flora and fauna of the environment become demons that can kill. Strict isolation is necessary. Also, there is the chance that the viability of the marrow cells may be reduced by handling. However, refinements in procedure are being made that give promise for better survival.

If the bone marrow replacement is successful, it gradually regains function. Its immune cells, red cells, and platelets are restored. With the cancer cells eliminated by the chemotherapy and radiation, the patient can return to good health.

Bioengineered Products of the Immune System

Some of the genes that code for the production of factors by cells of the immune system have been cloned. Consequently, these products can now be manufactured in large quantities for use in experimental cancer treatments. Some immunomodulators that are available include interferons, interleukin–2, tumor necrosis factor, colony-stimulating factors, and thymosin (Chapter 3). They enhance different aspects of the immune response. Not all substances work in all cancer patients, because cancer is actually a group of many different diseases. Some immune products are more effective against one form of the disease than another.

Unfortunately, serious side effects are associated with some immunostimulating drugs, when prescribed in pharmocological doses. Eventually, balanced concentrations of all the natural immune products will be used. As more become available, the aim is to duplicate the total innate resources of the body. By mimicking the body's own response, it is hoped we can eliminate the scourge of mankind forever.

Monoclonal Antibodies

Our ability to manufacture unlimited quantities of custommade antibodies, each specifically targeted at a person's tumor, has enormous therapeutic promise (Chapter 3). As technology improves, and the limitations of the procedure are overcome, its full potential in cancer treatment may be realized. New, innovative uses for monoclonals are constantly being introduced.

Vaccines

A vaccine may be prepared from the patient's own tumor cells. The cells are attenuated by radiation or by treatment with a chemotherapeutic agent, so they can no longer divide. They are inoculated into many different sites of the body, along with an immunostimulating agent like BCG. The rationale is that the attenuated cells, together with the nonspecific stimulator, will activate a larger portion of the immune capacity than is possible with the naturally developing tumor. There are various versions of this technique. One of these attempts to uncover concealed antigenic sites on the tumor cells by digesting away some of the surface. As the tumor markers become more visible to the immune system, their antigenicity may be increased.

Vaccination to protect against cancer is already a reality for newborn chicks. It prevents them from acquiring a tumor later in life, which had always proved very costly to the chicken industry. Chickens are susceptible to a lymphoma called Marek's disease. This widespread disorder has finally been brought under control with the vaccine which gives life-long lymphoma protection to chickens.

A commercial vaccine is also available to prevent feline leukemia. When used prophylactically, it prevents this lethal cancer from developing in cats. All cat owners are being advised to have their healthy pets vaccinated to protect them against leukemia.

Both Marek's disease and feline leukemia are caused by viruses. The antigenic determinants on the developing tumor cells are produced by the viruses themselves. When the attenuated vaccines are used, they prime or sensitize the immune cells of the healthy animal. The defenders become alert, waiting for the tumor to appear. A challenge by a tumor cell, at any time, results in a speedy and effective reprisal. The tumor cells are clobbered without delay, so they cannot multiply and outnumber the defense cells.

Vaccine preparation for other tumors is more difficult, since the TAAs are frequently variable. Some tumors contain several clones, each with different TAAs. This may be due to mutations that occur freely in aberrant cells. A heterogeneous population poses a formidable problem for the production of a single vaccine. It would have to be a mixture, capable of operating against each of the TAAs in a tumor mass.

With an increased understanding of the fundamental mechanisms of the immune response, we can expect imaginative new approaches to immunotherapy for cancer. Prophylactic, preventive vaccines against all human tumors have always been the dream of immunotherapists. As long as smallpox has been eradicated with a vaccine, why shouldn't we aim to do the same for cancer?

SUMMARY

One of the talents of the immune system is to recognize and destroy cancer cells when they appear. It is on guard at all times. When a tumor succeeds in gaining the upper hand, it is an indication of an outsmarted immune mechanism. The tactics of tumor cells to outdo their antagonists are cunning indeed.

Proof of the role of the immune system in tumor surveillance and containment comes from immunosuppressed patients. Immune suppression may be due to inborn errors, or it can be produced by chemicals, radiation, or life events. Whatever the cause, the incidence of tumors in suppressed individuals usually exceeds that of the normal population.

From animal experiments, we know that there is a genetic disposition to cancer. Some strains of mice have a higher incidence of certain types of tumors than others. Hereditary influences are also implicated in certain human cancers. This we cannot control. However, there are known environmental factors that are associated with an increased risk for some cancers. We can do something about these. Smoking can be eliminated, as well as excessive consumption of alcohol. The ultraviolet rays of the sun can be avoided, and asbestos needn't be inhaled. We can fight atmospheric pollution, and prevent stress with stress-modifying techniques. Foods that have carcinogenic potential can be shunned, and those that are associated with a reduction in cancer development can be included. There are many factors that are subject to our control which can have an important influence on the incidence of cancer.

A lengthy period of time may elapse between inception of a tumor and its clinical appearance. Frequently, the cause is so far removed from the effect, that it cannot even be associated with the disease. Therefore, it is important to be on guard at all times. We have the power to protect ourselves, and taking unnecessary chances does not pay off!

A strong immune system is the best insurance against cancer. In the future, medical examinations will have to include data on immunologic parameters, such as lymphocyte ratios, $T_H:T_S$, the phagocytic activity of macrophages and PMN leukocytes, NK cell number, serum concentrations of blocking antibodies to TAAs, and the level of thymic hormone in the serum. An immunologic appraisal can tell us what to expect. The values may identify those who are likely to experience disease. They can forewarn us to utilize all the knowledge we have accumulated about strengthening the immune system, to help it function effectively against cancer.

An improved understanding of cancer can increase a patient's confidence in dealing with his disease. Once the unknown is conquered, the panic and helplessness may be allayed and coping can become easier. New research is showing that anxiety and maladaptation cause stress, which can weaken the immune system. The physical and emotional pain of cancer can be devastating to the natural defenses. In fact, relaxation techniques are being used in many cancer centers to ease the strain of the disease, as well as the stressful effects of the treatments. The aim is to help revitalize the injured immune system to improve immune potential. It is hoped that the information in this chapter will assist in stemming the turbulence within the victim, frustrating the progress of his disease.

7

Protecting Your Immune System

The competing forces in nature have necessitated the development of our defense system. It contributes to a healthy and potentially long life. Of course, individual resistance varies, because who we are and how we live impinges on our well-being. The uniqueness of each person's immune system is determined by his genetic constitution, age, sex, and various life events. Such factors can influence ability to combat disease. The great protector may be abused with poor nutrition, physical or psychological stress, or hazardous environmental encounters. Its innate competency can be curtailed. We are becoming increasingly aware of the importance of a healthy life-style for a well-functioning immune system. To do a good job, it must have good support. Controlling the controllable factors in our lives is a personal responsibility for all of us.

The genes we inherit determine our ability to respond to different invading antigens. When living in closely knit groups, people frequently harbor the same germs. Yet, some come down with a disease, while others successfully evade it. One person may mobilize a good fight against one agent of disease, but respond feebly to another. There are high and low responders to individual antigens. These traits are genetically controlled.

We can't do much about genetic potential, age, or gender. However, we can take charge of the variables in everyday life, which may be risk factors. Understanding how immune responsiveness can be altered by diet, stress, radiation, immunosuppressive drugs, and various diseases should stimulate a protective instinct. It can improve your chances for living successfully and enjoying the good life.

Effect of Nutrition on the Immune Response

An individual's resistance to disease is influenced by his nutritional status. Nutrition also plays a significant role in recovery from disease. Severe protein deficiency causes a profound impairment of cell-mediated immunity (CMI). Many parts of the humoral system are also hurt. Even the nonspecific phagocytic cells can no longer kill efficiently when poorly nourished. The result is an increased susceptibility to infections, and a greater potential for tumor development.

Lymphocytes are highly active cells which are constantly dividing to produce clones. Many different clones are necessary, since each is capable of seeking out and responding to only one antigenic determinant on an invader. Adequate nutrition is needed to support the growth and multiplication of these large numbers of cells. In addition, some of the fully differentiated, nondividing immune cells function by means of substances they manufacture. The raw materials for their production can only be obtained from the daily intake of a variety of nutrients. To actively fight disease, large amounts of immunoglobulins, lymphokines, enzymes, and toxic oxidation products are produced. With inadequate nutrition, the manufacturing process is necessarily impaired, and immunodeficiency results.

In animal models for malnutrition studies, as well as in malnourished humans, the destruction of the immune apparatus is clearly evident. All the lymphoid organs shrink in size. The thymus gland (Figure 1-1) deteriorates rapidly and there is a decreased production of thymosin hormone. Immunoglobulin secretions are reduced. The titers of interferon and interleukin are diminished. Recruitment of phagocytes is hindered, and the activity of their enzymes, which degrade the pathogens, is weakened. Complement production is also altered. With no clearance of antigen-antibody complexes, the incidence of infectious diseases increases. So many parts of the defense network suffer that the immune system becomes virtually impotent and the pathogens can reign supreme.

Immune dysfunction due to malnutrition is most prevalent in underdeveloped countries. However, it is also a problem in affluent societies, among the critically ill and the elderly. Old people frequently eat poorly, due to loneliness, or the constant pain of degenerative diseases. Physiologic changes may contribute to a decreased appreciation of food. A reduction in physical activity, as well as medications, can also interfere with appetite. Some drugs obstruct the utilization of nutrients by the body, even though the diet is adequate. Alerting the physician to suspicious changes, before they continue too long, can help prevent deterioration of immune capacity.

In some cancer patients, there is poor absorption of nutrients, even though they are adequately taken in. Ironically, just when the defense system is needed most, it becomes debilitated by a lack of the raw materials that are needed to sustain it.

Young girls on weight-loss binges, who develop disorders like anorexia nervosa and bulimia nervosa, usually show reduced immune competence. Likewise, people on fad diets may suffer from a nutrient imbalance. They develop single nutrient deficiencies, which can inhibit susceptible members of the immune team. Maintaining normal immune function, with all the lymphocytes working at full capacity, requires a balance of nutrients.

The intake of massive doses of some dietary components can tax immune function. Recommended dietary allowances (RDA) have been established for many vitamins and minerals. They range from microgram to milligram quantities per day. There is no scientific evidence that intake, in excess of RDA, by healthy individuals is beneficial or safe.

Recently, a committee of scientists called on the Federal Food and Drug Administration (FDA) to initiate consumer protection measures for over-the-counter sales of vitamin and mineral supplements, since we do not know the long-term consequences of their daily use. When some isolated nutrients are consumed in large amounts, they can become toxic. Also, competition with other nutrients that are essential to the body is possible. A necessary substance may become depleted, because its absorption is prevented by large quantities of a supplement. Even if it is not harmful, consuming an unnecessary nutrient can be wasteful; when the tissues are saturated it is only eliminated. Sometimes, there is a danger that the body will become accustomed to megadoses of a vitamin. Then, if it must be stopped suddenly, a rebound deficiency can result.

Physicians are being urged to take patient histories about supplement use, and to document any toxic effects attributable to excessive doses. Vitamin abuse by healthy people, who self-prescribe to prevent disease, is finally arousing concern. It is always safer to include a variety of foods in the diet that are rich in the needed nutrients, since quantity is controllable, and balance is maintained.

The use of supplements should be reserved for conditions where specific deficiencies exist, as advised by health professionals. People with certain diseases may require supplements, as may food faddists who have become depleted of some essentials. Extras are frequently prescribed by the physician for pregnant and lactating women.

Overweight people who overeat suffer from infectious diseases more frequently than the normal population. Free, unused nutrients become available for bacterial growth. The bacteria thrive, and the immune system must work hard to combat them. The overwork can cause resistance to go down, while risk goes up.

Excess food consumption may also be a contributing factor for certain types of cancer. Insurance statistics have correlated overweight with an increased incidence of breast and colon cancers. They have been associated with fat intake. The major brunt of obesity is born by cell-mediated immunity (CMI) and the nonspecific system, both of which guard against cancer.

Rate of aging can be influenced by nutritional intervention. The life expectancy of experimental rats and mice were increased by moderate food restriction. Many physiologic processes of aging were retarded, as were the diseases that are usually associated with aging. It is not known whether similar interventions would be useful in humans, but statistics show that marked obesity has adverse effects on longevity.

Extremes are potential troublemakers. Too much or too little can exact a toll on the immune system. It is important to supply a variety of nutrients in moderation, so immune cells can live up to their genetic capabilities. Healthy people, on a varied diet, usually do not need extras. In this do-it-yourself era, variety, moderation, and balance should become the key words for food selection and proper nutrition.

Fortunately, immune suppression that is induced by poor nutrition is reversible. It may be corrected by consuming a wide variety of foods that assure adequate intake of all essential nutrients.

Dietary guidelines have been formulated by the Departments

of Agriculture and Health and Human Services for healthy people to stay healthy. They recommend selections from four major food groups, which are meant to be consumed in moderate amounts that maintain a desirable weight. (1) Meat group—choose from lean meats, poultry, dry beans, or fish. (2) Cereal group—select whole grain breads, cereals, rice, and corn. (3) Milk group—use low-fat milk products. (4) Vegetables and fruits—include green and yellow vegetables and citrus fruits. Fats should be limited to less than 30 percent of daily food intake, with near equal amounts of polyunsaturated, monounsaturated, and saturated forms. The rule of thumb is to eat less salt, sugar, and fat, but more fiber, which should be obtained from fruits and vegetables, as well as cereals and breads. Excessive amounts of any one nutrient should be avoided. If alcohol is consumed, it must be in moderation, since alcohol provides "empty calories" with no nutrient value.

Further information can be obtained free of charge by writing to: Human Nutrition Information Service, U.S. Department of Agriculture, Room 325A, Federal Building, Hyattsville, Maryland 20782.

The American Cancer Society has promulgated nutrition guidelines to identify possible cancer threats. They denounce diets that are high in fat and alcohol. Cured foods, that are prepared with smoke or nitrites, are labeled as possible cancer risks. Nitrites are used to develop the red color of processed meats. They can be converted to carcinogens by the acids of the stomach. Meticulous scrutiny of food labels is an important aspect of healthy eating.

EFFECT OF STRESS ON THE IMMUNE RESPONSE

Very often the mind becomes a partner with the body in determining health. Pressures that strain either the mind or body can cause stress. The common denominator of excessive physical or mental strain is the stress reaction. Nature has provided us with this method of coping in order to put the body into high gear, so it can deal effectively with danger or challenge. It is the familiar "fight or flight" reaction. However, if the system is activated persistently and intensely, without controls, nature's adaptation can become harmful. The immune system, as well as many other organs of the body suffer, thus increasing vulnerability to disease. Once you become aware of the destructive side of the stress reaction, the need to take control and harness it whenever possible should be obvious. Effective management of pressures and strains is an additional weapon in the struggle against disease.

The immediate physiologic effect of stress is the production of chemicals by the brain. A chain reaction is set up, as they stimulate an outpouring of hormones from the adrenal glands into the bloodstream (Figure 1–1). These secretions raise the blood sugar, thus providing more energy. The respiration rate increases to supply the additional demands of the body for oxygen. Blood pressure and heart function are escalated to circulate the sugar and oxygen quickly. The resources of the body are mobilized to handle the immediate danger.

The acute reaction can be readily demonstrated in experiments with unstressed mice. When injected with adrenal hormones, all the physiologic effects of true stress are mimicked. At the same time, the toll on the lymphoid organs is great; they decrease in size. There is also a pronounced destruction of lymphocytes, and nonspecific phagocytes are depressed.

Slowing down the immune system during an emergency is nature's intention. Survival is favored by concentrating all the body's resources for fighting, or escaping from the immediate danger. Energy that would normally be required for an inflammatory reaction to respond to a wound which may be suffered in the melee is conserved. The immune system is put on hold.

When there is excessive or prolonged triggering of the stress reaction due to physical or mental causes, the adrenal glands are forced to work at peak capacity. The same inhibition of immune defenses results as occurs in a time of emergency. Susceptibility to disease can follow.

In mice afflicted with tumors, the tumor volume can be made to increase by subjecting the animals to stress. The normal checks on the tumor by immune cells are diminished. This can be duplicated with injections of adrenal hormones, without the stress. The numbers of natural killer (NK) cells and macrophages that operate against the tumor are decreased. The inappropriate triggering of stress can upset the normal balances of the body, increasing vulnerability.

In humans, the injection of some adrenal hormones causes a prompt reduction in lymphocyte number in the blood, and a rapid shrinkage of the thymus gland. The decrease in T lymphocytes is greater than B. The loss is due mainly to a decrease in T_H number. Since T_H is the pivotal cell, which is involved in the normal activities of most of the immune network, its loss is detrimental to protection (Figure 2–3). The number of suppressor T cells (T_S) that remains is greater than T_H. The high ratio of T_S to T_H favors immune suppression, and furthers the decrease in immune power.

The reduction in available lymphocytes is temporary in humans, and not due to cell destruction, as in mice. The circulating lymphocytes are merely redistributed. They are forced back into the lymph nodes and bone marrow. When the stress-related chemicals are used up, there is a return to normal.

The usual activities of human phagocytes are also altered by stress hormones. Ravenous appetites of "big eaters" and PMNs are dulled, inhibiting efficient ingestion of intruders. Those that are caught are not readily degraded, because the enzymes are impaired.

Unbridled stress, which invokes oversecretion of hormones, stifles both the nonselective, first line of defense, as well as the selective follow-up defenders. The scene is set for a successful takeover by disease. Sometimes the disease is due to a virus which has been lying dormant in the body for a long time. It becomes activated when the body's favorable balance is upset by stress.

The effect of poor stress management is frequently seen in students at exam time, when stress hormones deplete the available immune cells. Ironically, a cold develops just at the crucial time, when it is important to be in good condition. Or, an illness which has been on the mend will become exacerbated. Skin eruptions are also a by-product of test-taking. The ever-present bacteria on the skin seize their opportunity as soon as stress hormones become plentiful, and immune activity declines. Acne results.

Trench mouth (Vincent's infection) is frequently associated with excessive stress in students. It is an acute bacterial attack on the tissues surrounding the teeth. The opportunistic pathogens are normal inhabitants of the mouth that are usually kept in check. They pounce when defenses are down. The condition can be aggravated by poor health habits, such as faulty nutrition, eating highly spiced foods, smoking, and alcohol abuse.

Secretion of adrenal hormones is always increased by depression; despair evokes the stress reaction. The severity of the resulting immune impairment depends on how long the depression persists. This was demonstrated in studies of individuals who recently suffered the death of a close family member. Bereavement was chosen for study, because it is frequently responsible for a state of persistent depression and stress. As predicted, grief resulted in a decreased lymphocyte count. There was also a decrease in natural killer activity and in interferon (IF) production. In some family members, the poor immune response lasted as long as 14 months following the death. This is a dangerously long time to suffer impaired defenses, since most of the ingredients necessary to ward off infection and cancer are in short supply during this period. Depression can increase the risk for medical problems.

Psychological stress affects the entire body, not only the immune system. It can cause you to gain weight you don't need, or lose weight you can't afford. It depletes powers of concentration, causes tension headaches, and may contribute to ulcers, heart disease, fatigue, and exhaustion. As long as you are aware of the damages caused by stress, it should serve as an incentive to avoid destructive behavior, and build stress resistance. This takes perseverance and hard work, since the negative component of behavior must be replaced with positive attitudes.

Physical stress also needs to be regulated. Not getting enough sleep, constant pain, sudden chilling or overheating, noise, and air pollution all contribute to the buildup of the reaction. Drugs can also be interpreted as stress by a body that is not accustomed to them. The accumulation of pressures, even some we may not be aware of, can take a toll on the immune system. Some factors that can modify the effects of the stress reaction are easy to monitor; they include good nutrition, adequate exercise, and rest.

Since stress drains the body of its energy reserves, well-balanced meals are important. Also, try to spend at least half an hour at physical exercise that is noncompetitive, several days a week. It will help blow off steam, and relax the mind, as well as strengthen the body. Fitness promotes an easier recovery from the stress reaction, and makes you look better, too. Adequate rest can contribute to a sense of well-being and an ability to cope. It can increase resistance to stress.

Don't brood about situations that are beyond your control. Handle stressful events with a philosophical attitude. Keep on top of things. Lose yourself in work or recreation, until you find a way to master the stressful problem. Try to come up with constructive solutions quickly, in order to prevent the destructive effects of prolonged stress. Learn from mistakes which resulted in stress, and try to prevent them the next time.

Some people are able to deal with the pressures of life better than others. They overcome reverses quickly, and prevent the damaging effects of stress. For those who don't cope well, there are published techniques for relaxation and meditation which can help control stress. They should be used in everyday life. When stress is properly managed, a sense of well-being and calm prevails. The immune system is given the chance to function at full capacity.

Many hospitals are recognizing the negative effects of stress on the healing process, and have taken measures to control them. They are utilizing relaxation programs at the bedside to protect the immune system, and to enhance its healing powers. The techniques of faith and serenity are serving as support mechanisms for medicine. The outcome is encouraging.

Occupational fitness and mental health programs are being offered to employees by many large companies. They focus on stress counseling. The programs are designed to alleviate tensions in the workplace, and to make people aware of their unyielding behavior. They deal with stress-related disorders that can affect production. The emphasis is on improvement of behavior and life-style, to eliminate extreme responses to difficult situations. A pleasant outlook, and the conscious control of feelings of pressure and time urgency can reduce the stress syndrome. Companies using these programs find that expenditures for health care due to absenteeism, accidents, and benefit claims have decreased, while productivity increases. The link between mental health and body health is finally being recognized.

A new discipline has recently been introduced to medical science, psychoneuroimmunology (PNI). It is based on the premise that thoughts and emotional state can alter the immune system. It is being tested in experimental groups of cancer patients, who are taught relaxation techniques and guided imagery, to go along with their conventional chemotherapy treatments. The aim is to mobilize and enhance the body's immune fight against the cancer. It is also being tried on the healthy elderly to prevent cancer, since immune function declines with age, and the cancer rate is increased.

Opponents challenge the idea that outlook can alter the prognosis for cancer, although they agree that it can favorably affect the ability to cope. It can lessen the mental shock of the dreaded disease, and reduce the hormones associated with despair.

There are some conditions where adrenal hormones are helpful, and they are used pharmaceutically. Advantage is taken of their suppressive effects on lymphocytes, in cases where the immune system overreacts, or its normal action needs to be squelched. Cortisols or their derivatives are prescribed to prolong the survival of grafts in transplant recipients. They delay graft rejection. They also alleviate the angry immune responses in autoimmune diseases. Acute inflammatory conditions are reduced, allergic reactions are moderated, and lymphocyte numbers are decreased in lymphocytic cancers. They are usually prescribed for a limited time, since undesirable side effects can develop.

The adrenal hormones are powerful chemicals, that can serve as friend or foe, depending on the condition. Understanding how they function and interact in the body can help to control the stress cascade and harness it for maximum benefit.

HEALTH EFFECTS OF EXERCISE

Moderate physical activity can improve the well-being of both body and mind. It can enhance the physique, reduce stress, and increase powers of concentration. The result is a positive effect on the immune response. All people are being advised to remain physically active throughout life, regardless of age.

In our aging society, the health benefits of exercise for the elderly are being emphasized. Seniors need regular exercise to preserve body function and prolong independent living. Although there is a normal decline in aerobic capacity with age, it is frequently slowed down by safe, habitual conditioning programs. There are economic benefits, too, since the usual high cost of health services for the aged can be reduced as a result of active living.

Physical exercises that are tailored to the needs of the individual should be practiced on a regular basis. The recommendation is one half-hour, at least three times per week. Once scheduled into the routine, it is not too difficult to maintain. The exercises can increase endurance, muscle strength, and flexibility, as well as protect against the damaging effects of too much stress hormone that persists in the body too long. Planned fitness programs are a good way of having fun, while keeping fit. However, everything must be done gradually and in moderation, because you can't get into shape all at once.

On the other hand, physical activity which leads to exhaustion can be stressful. This is frequently encountered in competitions, where athletes push themselves to the limits of capacity, to beat the clock and to achieve records. The body responds with the adrenal stress hormones, which have their usual negative effects on the immune system. If continued over a long period of time, the competitor can fall prey to the ravages of disease. An innocuous virus, which is ordinarily only a nuisance, can become a lethal virus, due to an overstressed immune system. Viral infections of the respiratory tract are seen more commonly in athletes at the end of a training period, as compared to the start, since there is a buildup of fatigue. The T lymphocyte is dramatically depleted by exhaustive exercise. The normal ratio of $T_H:T_S$ cells decreases. With low T_H levels, the entire immune network is impaired (Figure 2–3), and both humoral immunity and CMI suffer. The concentration of protective antibodies in the respiratory secretions and saliva is significantly decreased. The NK cell count is also depleted. The drop in cell number lasts for about 24 hours after a period of exertion, and then gradually returns to normal levels when the strain is relieved. Sustained, intense exercise that hurts results in delayed recovery, and is not conducive to good immune function.

Continued enthusiasm for competition, in spite of detrimental experiences, is attributed to a pain-relieving chemical produced by the brain. It is believed to be responsible for enabling the athlete to keep going, in spite of the body's exhaustion. It is a brain opioid, capable of inducing a sense of well-being, which is commonly known as the "runner's high." It masks the pain, which should be the signal to stop. With no brakes, the competitor frequently pushes on until collapse. Measurements of brain opioids, secreted into the blood of runners who continued on until collapse, were found to be approximately four times greater than in those who did not break down.

In some people, stressful exercise can cause exercise-induced rhinitis, a nasal congestion, or exercise-induced bronchospasm (EIB) and asthma (EIA). Rapid increased oral breathing brings cold air directly into the lungs. There is no time for the usual warming or moistening of the air by the nasal passages. When unprocessed air contacts the delicate lung tissues, there is a drop in temperature and drying of the airways. Such an irritation may produce a physical allergy. Released histamine and other mediators have been implicated. It is believed they are secreted from storage depots in the mast cells of the lungs. They contribute to airway constriction, wheezing, coughing, and gasping for breath. The episode is self-limiting when the cause is removed.

A warm-up period before exercising helps to reduce the incidence of exercise-induced bronchospasm. It should consist of calisthenics or light running before the more strenuous exercise that follows.

The EIA condition has only recently been recognized as an immune response. Coaches are being alerted to screen for EIA among competitors for sports events and college athletes who apply for teams. Questionnaires that help diagnose the condition are becoming part of the history-taking practice. An applicant must reveal if he needs to stop and catch his breath after running one half mile. There are questions like, "If you ran one mile, then sat 10 or 15 minutes, would you find it increasingly difficult to breathe?" This would indicate a progressive allergic reaction, starting with mast cell irritation, then histamine release, and finally asthmatic constriction. Other questions are, "While resting, would your chest feel tight? Would you cough?" The screening program also includes exercise challenge.

International medical athletic committees have approved the use of specific drugs for EIA to counteract the mediators of mast cells. Once diagnosed, EIA can be successfully managed, as evidenced by the medals won by Olympians who have been diagnosed with the condition. The tendency for several members of the same family to suffer with EIA has been documented.

The stress effects of exhaustive exercise can be prevented by the gradual development of aerobic fitness. Although adrenal stress hormones are also produced in aerobically trained individuals, the length of time they remain in the blood is decreased. They are more transient in the aerobically fit, and return to baseline levels more rapidly.

Extremes are always associated with risk. Not enough exercise, as well as too much, are both hazardous. Lifelong moderate exercise can prolong active life, and enhance its quality. All is not lost, however, if the training didn't start in youth. There are data that show the beneficial effects of habitual exercise started at an advanced age. Physical decline attributed to aging may be slowed at any time by regular exercise.

EFFECT OF ALCOHOL

Alcohol is just as threatening to immune defenses as other stressors. It stimulates the release of adrenal hormones, as in the typical stress reaction. Prolonged use can result in depletion of immune function. Clinical studies have shown a pronounced susceptibility to infection in alcoholics, and an increased risk for cancer. This is due to the generalized breakdown in health that usually accompanies chronic alcoholism, as well as the specific inhibition of immune function. PMNs, which are a first line of defense against invaders, are decreased in number. Those that remain respond sluggishly when confronted with a pathogen. Macrophage mobilization and phagocytosis is also suppressed. The nonspecific immune system is hurt. Fortunately, its normal response gradually returns when abstinence is maintained.

The specific arm of the defense system is also altered by persistent alcohol challenge. A marked defect in T- and B-cell regulation results, which leads to immune suppression. Pathogens find it easy to gain a foothold and multiply.

An alcoholic habit is frequently used to escape a stressful problem. The problem can't disappear, because intelligent coping is prevented. Alcohol merely compounds the stress reaction, and increases the risk for new problems with disease.

EFFECT OF ENVIRONMENTAL RADIATION

Breathing clean air is our fundamental right. It needs to be protected, because good health depends upon good air. Exposure to pollutants can cause injuries that may be immediate or delayed. It is important to take control of each breath to decrease risks.

One of the most dangerous forms of contamination that is despoiling our planet is radiation. It is an invisible peril that causes insidious and progressive damage to all forms of life. Although natural environmental radiation is everpresent and unavoidable, additional man-induced emissions have to be controlled. Radiation that escapes accidentally during the commercial production of nuclear energy, and the ionized particles from exploding nuclear weapons are equally damaging. An understanding of how life on earth is being threatened should arouse public fears and concern.

Exposure to high levels of radiation causes radiation sickness. The pathological effects may occur soon after exposure, or there may be a delayed disease process, even many years later. The magnitude of the damage depends on the intensity of radiation received. Radiation sickness from high doses can kill within a few hours. The entire body is affected, since there are multiple direct hits. Highly active cells, those which are constantly dividing are the most severely injured. Many of their vital components become inactivated.

Since cell division is a major characteristic of all bone marrow cells, the elements of the blood and immune system suffer most. Red blood cell formation is inhibited, which results in anemia. A decrease in blood clotting factors favors hemorrhaging. Clone formation is inhibited, so CMI and antibody synthesis are impaired. The nonspecific cells of the immune system become inept, since phagocytosis is diminished. If the patient doesn't die, he suffers the consequences of a crippled immune capacity.

Other body parts also suffer. The gastrointestinal lining disintegrates, since it is composed of dividing cells that normally renew themselves. Loss of appetite, nausea, vomiting, and diarrhea result. Later, cancers of the gastrointestinal tract abound. Reproductive cells are highly vulnerable, since they are in a state of cell division. Sterility is a frequent outcome of radiation damage. The developing fetus in a pregnant woman is susceptible, since it is constantly increasing in size and making more cells. Exposed fetuses that survive have a high incidence of cancer. Excessive radiation can produce a constellation of devastating events.

If radiation damage doesn't kill, cell repair is initiated soon after the hit. However, the repair may not be 100 percent effective. The injury can be magnified if repeat exposures occur, since radiation doses are cumulative and have a linear dose-response relationship. It is important to evacuate immediately, in the event of a nuclear disaster, so cells are given the chance to heal themselves. The extent of the radiation injury depends on the time span over which it is absorbed, as well as the dose received.

Lesser doses of radiation can also kill, but it takes a longer time, even many years. Only one particle in a cell may be bombarded with radiation. It becomes ionized, acquiring an electric charge, which enables it to react with other particles in the cell to initiate toxic reactions. A chain of events is started gradually causing secondary ionizations throughout the cell. The cumulative damage wreaks havoc. The cell becomes crippled and may eventually die.

Radiation damage that alters the genes within cells can cause cancers. They show up in months or even many years after exposure. Leukemia is most prevalent, but other forms of cancer also occur. In the survivors of Hiroshima and Nagasaki, cancers of the thyroid gland, breast, and lungs were numerous; some took as long as 20 years to appear. The incidence was inversely proportional to the distance from the center of exposure, since it is dose-dependent.

It is predicted that the Russian nuclear accident at Chernobyl will affect people for many years to come. Officials of international agencies for radiological protection estimate that thousands of people, perhaps up to one-half million, will die of radiation-induced cancers arising from that disaster.

The late effects of nonlethal doses of radiation may become manifested in perpetuity. They involve changes in the genes of reproductive cells, the carriers of our heritage. There may be a direct hit to a gene in an egg or sperm, or the gene may become damaged by a sequential reaction, started in another part of the cell. Mutations can result which show up as defective offspring.

The disastrous effects of radiation can be transmitted for generations to come. What a legacy to hand down to our children!

Protective measures are advised that can lessen inhalation of radioactive particles. Immediately following a radiation accident, the nose and mouth should be covered with several layers of damp cloth to serve as a mask. A shelter can also reduce the inhaled dose. Windows, doors, and ventilation systems must be tightly shut. It is essential to identify and reject contaminated food and water. Safe and speedy evacuation should be planned.

The particular radioactive elements that are produced by the nuclear event determine which organs will be affected most. Different chemical elements are attracted to different parts of the body. Some home into the bones, others build up in the liver or spleen, while some are picked up by the thyroid gland. Wherever they are, they all emit radiation and do the same type of damage.

So far, we have no simple, practical treatments for large-scale radiation exposure. Only the thyroid gland can be protected, by supplying the gland with iodine before an expected encounter. Since iodine is a normal requirement of the gland, feeding supplemental doses beforehand causes it to become saturated. Then, when exposed to the radioactive iodine, it has no need for anymore. The FDA has approved the use of potassium iodide to be prescribed for radiation emergencies. The protection is limited to the thyroid gland; other organs are not safeguarded.

Treatment with antibiotics controls the infections due to a depressed immune system. For destroyed bone marrow, transplants are possible, but they present many dangerous problems of matching, unless a healthy identical twin is available. Experience with bone marrow transplants in the Chernobyl accident suggests that the benefits are limited. And what about the dilemma of sterility, the damaged young, and later cancers?

At the present time, prevention is our best weapon against

radiation. The radioactivity in the earth and its atmosphere is steadily increasing. Nobody knows how to eliminate it. Someday, we may lose our right to drink its water, plant in its soil, and breathe its air. Shouldn't we all take up the vigil, and speak out on the health effects of environmental hazards? Political clout is needed to insure a safe planet. It is a critical public health issue that involves all of us. We must become the guardians of our earth, in order to lessen genetic abnormalities, cancer, and the curtailment of the life span.

Just as the perils of intentional, man-made radiation are increasingly becoming a public issue, attention to the natural sources of emission are also intensifying. Radon gas from the earth is making its way into homes, and is causing much concern.

Radon is a radioactive gas, which is a breakdown product of uranium, a natural element in rock and soil. It is present in different concentrations, in different locations, on our planet. Radon gas from decaying uranium seeps into buildings through open joints and cracks in foundations and walls. The water supply may also become contaminated. Monitoring radon in the home is becoming big business, since lung cancer is clearly associated with this invisible and odorless gas. It was first recognized as a hazard in uranium miners, and then experiments with laboratory animals confirmed the lung cancer effects. Malignancy is proportional to radon exposure. The Centers for Disease Control (CDC) estimates that as many as 12 million homes may have unacceptable radon levels. They can be found in nearly every state.

The measures needed to remove the threat of radon from the home depend on the extent of the problem and where it is localized. It can involve major renovations, such as digging up contaminated areas within and around the foundation when high emissions are evident, or the solution may be simple. Frequently, it can be corrected by improving ventilation, better insulation, or sealing joints and cracks. Guidelines and standards have been published for new construction which can make homes radon-resistant.

The ozone layer of the upper atmosphere is also a cause for concern, since a progressive depletion is being monitored. The damage can be seen in the Antarctic in the form of an ever-increasing hole. Ozone normally absorbs harmful ultraviolet radiation from the sun, thus shielding all life on earth. As bigger and bigger holes are developing in the ozone, more radiation is reaching the earth. If unchecked, the immune system can become one of the numerous casualties of the increased radiation.

Chemists are implicating man-made chemicals, the chlorofluorocarbons (CFCs) and halons that contain bromine as the threat to the ozone layer. They accumulate high above the earth where they are bombarded with ultraviolet radiation from the sun. Chlorine and bromine are released, which combine with ozone and destroy it. These chemicals are used commercially as fire suppressants, solvents, propellants in spray cans, refrigerants, and in the manufacture of foam products for insulation and packaging materials.

Controlling the manufacture of CFCs and halons has become a political and economic issue. International conferences have been organized to establish treaties that will limit future production of these ozone-destroying chemicals throughout the globe. Taking preventive measures now could eliminate future biological grief to all living things, animals and plants.

EFFECT OF SEX HORMONES

There isn't much we can do about gender, but information about sex hormones can help in understanding their relationship to immunologic processes. Hormones can interact in diverse ways with the immune system.

Most females enjoy immunological superiority. The female sex hormone, estrogen, appears to be responsible for an enhanced immune response in many mammalian species. In males, the immune response is less active after puberty, when the male hormones increase.

Most of the experiments designed to determine the effects of sex hormones were done with mice. In certain strains, both castrated males and normal females were found to make higher concentrations of antibodies in response to antigens than normal males. When antigens are used that stimulate CMI, specifically, the same superior response is obtained. Both the humoral system and CMI benefit from physiologic concentrations of estrogen. The thymus gland is more active in these groups, indicating a positive effect of estrogen on thymic cell function. On the other hand, in experiments where the estrogen is injected, high concentrations can inhibit the immune system.

Progesterone, another female sex hormone, has the opposite effect on immune power. It is synthesized in the second half of the menstrual cycle, and is also present in large amounts during pregnancy. Progesterone causes a reduction in the number of T_H cells, and its action is dose-dependent. The high concentration during pregnancy together with elevated estrogen levels, enables the mother's immune system to tolerate the fetus. From an immunological point of view, the fetus may be considered as a foreign graft, since half of its determinants are inherited from the father. These are necessarily foreign to the mother, and theoretically, the fetus should be rejected. The depressed state of the T_H cells due to the hormones of pregnancy may play a significant role in tolerance of the fetus. At the same time, normal resistance to many diseases is reduced during pregnancy. The infinite wisdom of evolution has evolved a stable state by intermittently providing estrogen and progesterone during the normal cycle to balance each other. Survival of the species depends on both hormones.

Male sex hormones stimulate suppressor T lymphocytes. With enhanced T_s activity, the pivotal T_H cell is inhibited and the humoral and cell mediated immune responses are decreased.

This was demonstrated by injecting the male hormone, testosterone, into certain strains of castrated male mice. They suffered a reduced response to viral infections and other antigens. The action was concentration-dependent.

Testosterone has also been used in experiments with chicks. B lymphocytes can be prevented from developing in the young animal merely by dipping the fertilized egg into a solution of testosterone for a few minutes. Without B cells, there are no plasma cells, and consequently no antibody formation.

Sex hormones have been studied in relation to autoimmune diseases, where angry, destructive immune responses are made to self determinants. It seemed unusual that such diseases should predominate in females. For example, systemic lupus erythematosus (SLE) affects ten females to every male. When oral contraceptives are used that contain estrogen, the condition worsens. On the other hand, removal of the ovaries, to deprive the body of estrogens, calms the disease process. In both males and females with SLE, above normal titers of estrogen have been demonstrated in the blood. A possible explanation is the enhancement of T_H activity by estrogen. Unwanted antibody formation is increased in autoimmune-prone females during the estrogen phase of the cycle.

Experiments with certain strains of mice have shown that castrated males resemble females who suffer accelerated autoimmune diseases. Suppression of the condition can be accomplished by injections of testosterone. The testosterone stimulates suppressor T lymphocytes, which slow down the destructive T_H response against self antigens.

EFFECT OF AGE

Immune capacity changes with age. It is lowest in the very young and the very old. Both antibody response and CMI decline markedly with advancing years. At the same time, autoantibodies frequently develop in the elderly. The passage of time also causes the accessory phagocytic cells and complement to become sluggish and inefficient. This results in an increase of circulating immune complexes, which are not removed efficiently. The ability to combat cancer and infections becomes seriously compromised without an alert first line and second line of defense.

The role of the immune system in influencing longevity was documented in a continuous study of a healthy human population until the time of death of each participant. Within 3 years prior to demise, there was a significant decrease in lymphocyte number. These lowered blood counts were independent of both the age at the time of death, and cause of death. A physiological stress is implicated which depresses the lymphocyte number, and may be responsible for the final event. The triggering stresses have not been identified.

Chronological age is not synonymous with physiologic or functional age. The organs and tissues of some individuals weather more rapidly than others. Some of the decline associated with age, is influenced by life-style. It is possible to hold back the ravages of time with healthful choices: the food you eat, the stress you avoid, and maintaining physical fitness. These can all contribute to feelings of well-being in a senior.

Immune response as well as mental outlook can benefit from good health practices. In fact, many life insurance companies are planning to cut their losses by promoting healthful living. They are proposing lower rates for policy holders who exercise on a regular basis, who don't smoke, and control weight and stress. Perhaps economic incentives will help to keep people from killing themselves!

Sensible, moderate living is the key to a good quality of life. It is important to take charge of your own health by steering the everyday controllable factors. It is not possible to delegate this responsibility to professionals, because no one can be as interested or involved as you with the intricacies of yourself.

SUMMARY

Taking control of your well-being can enhance immune responses and contribute to a good quality of life. Encounters that normally occur during a lifetime impinge on a preset immune capacity. They are the modifying factors that can enhance or reduce the potential you were born with.

Dietary habits are an important modulator, with a direct influence on the cells of the immune system. These are active cells, constantly utilizing the energy you supply. The products they produce are only as good as the raw materials offered. Without proper nutrition, immune cells cannot perform their function to produce antibodies and other secretions. In addition, immune cells depend on clone formation to function effectively against intruders that encroach on health. To produce whole armies from a single cell requires a variety of balanced nutrients. The balance is delicate, so it is not only what you eat that counts, but how much of each food. Experiments have shown that both under-and overnutrition are detrimental to the immune system. It is important to keep moderation and balance in mind, and resist those fad diets that suggest a limited number of foods. Imbalances cannot supply the needs of an army that fights valiantly moment by moment of every day.

Stress is another modulator that can undermine immune competence. Increasingly, it is being associated with many illnesses; it is a harbinger of disease. Some stresses are easy to control, while others are the result of life events that are difficult to handle. As long as we understand the detrimental effects of stress, it should be an incentive to cope better, in order to diminish the potential for harm to the immune system. Behavioral techniques that work to minimize stress are becoming important tools in medicine. The healing power of the mind is finally being recognized.

Aerobic fitness can also influence immune capacity. Although trained individuals make an adrenal response to stress, the hormones are rapidly depleted when the reaction ceases. The faster they are removed from the body, the less the harm that is inflicted on immune cells. On the other hand, excessive, sustained, and exhausting physical exercise serves as a stressor that stimulates the release of large amounts of adrenal hormones. For best results, exercise should be tailored to the needs of the individual in a fitness program. Gradual conditioning makes you feel better about yourself, and can be beneficial to your immune apparatus. Even the physical decline associated with aging may be retarded with exercise training.

Alcoholics put themselves at risk for many diseases since alcohol interferes with the normal defense against invaders. The effectiveness of all arms of the immune system is diminished. Fortunately, it is never too late to change. The immune response can gradually recuperate when it is no longer bombarded with the toxin.

Radiation is detrimental to actively dividing cells. The bone marrow, which is the place of origin of immune cells and other elements of the blood, is among the most seriously hurt. An understanding of the damage that radiation imposes on the immune system should incite people to demand protection from man-induced radiation, as well as natural radiation hazards. Prevention is our best weapon, so far, to protect against the devastating effects, since medicine cannot adequately correct the damage inflicted. A joint effort is needed to voice concern about radiation protection.

8

AIDS

The Late Twentieth-Century Disaster

Acquired immunodeficiency syndrome (AIDS) is a new disease that has suddenly descended upon us. Most of its victims are doomed; more than half have died so far. Only a small percentage live longer than 3 years after diagnosis. Where AIDS came from, nobody knows for sure. That it is here to stay is pretty much certain, because the number of casualties continues to rise each year. It is spread by a virus that is found in body fluids, especially in blood and semen. In the United States, men with high-risk sexual life-styles were the first to be associated with the disease. They are homosexuals or bisexuals with multiple partners. Gradually, the virus is also infiltrating their heterosexual contacts. Intravenous drug users, who share unsterilized needles, succumb readily to the voracious virus. Their numbers predominate among heterosexual victims. Even children are not exempt, since the disease is transmitted from afflicted pregnant mothers to their newborn. Transfusion recipients and organ transplant patients were at high risk before mandatory testing for AIDS.

Once the victim is infected, there is no way to shake the virus. It becomes incorporated into the genes, and persists forever. AIDS has become a public health problem, which is barely responding so far to measures taken to contain it. The potential for a major disaster can be compared to the devastations of the historic plagues.

The disease causes a progressive immune dysfunction, so that the victim is stripped of all natural defenses. He is left unarmed to do battle with a hostile environment that harbors bacteria, viruses, fungi, and all sorts of lowly parasites. Cancer, too, becomes a threat. The virus is able to evade natural immune defenses by integrating itself into the genic structure of host cells. No drugs are available to permanently conquer the virus, or to restore the injured immune system. To date, there is no preventive vaccine, and no medical technique to stem the progression of the plague. The only effective countermeasure at the present time is widespread education, to teach awareness of the disease and behavior modification. The individual's power to protect himself is greater than any therapeutic measures offered by medical science so far.

In the days before the educational campaigns were launched, high-risk behavior was fashionable in certain groups. The pretty coed, G. S., became a victim. She was a serious student at a large urban college. The demands of classes occupied most of her time, and precluded an active social life. For 2 years she resisted the Thursday night parties which were a ritual in the dorm. However, when her roommate hosted a get-together far into the night, she had no choice but to walk in on the celebration of Thursday. She remembered that the air was polluted with the sweet smell of smoke. Everyone was carefree and casual, never showing any concern for the consequences of their actions. The murky air, peer pressure, and the desire to build self-esteem all joined forces to undo her reserve. She recited the events of that fateful night, in response to questions by the resident assigned to her care, in an isolation room of the city hospital.

After smoking pot, G. S. started to experiment with intravenous drugs. The incentive was always to promote an image. Soon after graduation, her career was successfully launched in the field of her major. As confidence soared, there was no longer any need for risky behavior. She was able to abstain. Now, 5 years after graduation, the pretty twenty-seven-year-old lay dying of AIDS; the price of Thursday.

At first, she refused to summon her parents, who lived in another state. However, as the pain-filled days merged mercilessly, and death was almost upon her, G. S. agreed to calling them. They arrived in the hospital room, uninformed as to their daughter's ailment. As soon as the diagnosis was revealed, both parents reacted by turning around and walking out. AIDS is a social problem, as well as a medical dilemma.

Unlike many other viral diseases, AIDS is not transmitted by ordinary contacts. It is fragile when outside the body, so droplets in the air from sneezes and coughs that may contain viruses are not infectious. Associations through the household setting do not make you vulnerable. The evidence comes from numerous studies of family members close to AIDS patients. None of the household investigations in the United States or in Africa have demonstrated infection by ordinary contact. It is transmitted mainly through blood and semen. Precautions must be taken in disposing of such infectious wastes. Instruments or appliances, like needles or shavers, that may become contaminated with the blood of an AIDS patient must be avoided. The virus can be inactivated by heat, freshly diluted bleach, peroxide, alcohol, and Lysol.

The victims in the United States are mostly males. They are cut down early in life, usually in their twenties to fifties. Gradually the virus is spreading to women, too, through heterosexual contacts and intravenous drug abuse. The efficiency of transmission appears to be greater from men to women than vice-versa. Epidemiological data suggest that contact with female prostitutes is a significant source of female-to-male transmission.

Since the stigma associated with this tragic disease is devastating, the tainted frequently become isolated from friends and family, in a time of greatest need. Psychological trauma can develop because of confusion and uncertainty about the disease. Economically, too, the victim becomes an outcast. Humiliations about money arise, when it is no longer possible to hold a job. This is compounded by discrimination against AIDS patients by many insurance companies. Those who are still able to work usually face prejudices in the workplace, in health facilities, and even at home. Widespread fears concerning contagion by casual contact abound. Even at the very end, many morticians are refusing to handle the bodies for embalming. A panic-stricken public is reacting vehemently to the disease.

HIV

The culprit is human immunodeficiency virus (HIV). It infiltrates a victim from infected blood, semen, or vaginal secretions. Once inside, it makes use of several types of body cells to entrench itself.

The macrophage serves as an important settling place. It is the large phagocytic cell of the immune system, which is alert to most intruders. Normally, it engulfs trespassers and clobbers them with stored enzymes and toxic chemicals. But not HIV; the virus is resistant to the usual poisons. It can live comfortably inside macrophages without being killed and without killing its host. The macrophage is taken captive by HIV. To keep itself busy, the parasite makes more viruses. The macrophage houses the progeny and serves as a repository. It contributes to the persistence of the virus. Since many macrophages are mobile, the deadly cargo is soon spread all over the body. Infected, viable macrophages can be obtained from the blood, lungs, bone marrow, and brains of most victims. The laden macrophages are believed to participate in the destruction of brain cells.

The helper T lymphocyte (T_H) is also a homing place for HIV. It has receptors on its surface that fasten to the virus. HIV can invade T_H cells directly, or the virus may be presented to the lymphocytes by macrophages that house them. Unlike the macrophages, T_H cannot adjust to the intruder's presence. As the virus replicates, T_H becomes incapacited and soon dies. A check of the blood count can reveal the depletion of T_H cells. This is one of the diagnostic signs of AIDS.

Without T_H, which is the pivotal cell of the immune network, many of the other components of the system are left stranded and unable to function normally. Activity is altered in all types of T cells, B cells, NK, and macrophages, since they all depend on T_H. Life-threatening infections result, which are characteristic of AIDS.

Rectal and colon cells also bear receptors that can bind HIV. The virus is able to multiply in invaded cells, and progeny are released for many weeks after infection. The rectal cells can serve as a route for infiltration. From here, the virus can spread to immune cells, and eventually to the brain.

As the virus continues to replicate, some progeny are shed into body fluids, including blood, saliva, seminal fluid (bathes sperm), tears, urine, breast milk, spinal fluid, and vaginal secretions. Enough virus for transmission is present mainly in blood, semen, and vaginal mucus. The concentration in other fluids is much lower.

Genesis of HIV

Pinpointing the place of origin of the virus has led to much speculation and debate. It has become a point of contention between countries, and is responsible for resentments, and accusations of prejudice and racism.

In some scientific reports, central Africa has been implicated as the source. Others refute this hypothesis, claiming there is not enough evidence. The World Health Organization is taking a noncommittal position, calling the origin of the virus a continuing mystery.

Evidence that associates Africa with the virus comes from blood serum obtained from healthy African children, which was routinely preserved. The blood had been drawn for a variety of tests in the 1950s and 1960s. Approximately 65 percent of these samples tested positive for the AIDS virus, using the antibody test that is now employed to help diagnose the disease. Positive tests were not obtained with similarly preserved sera from other areas.

In addition, many African green monkeys harbor a virus which is similar to HIV. About half the monkeys tested so far have produced antibodies to the monkey virus. Infected animals remain healthy, possibly because the virus is strongly immunogenic in its primate host, and is contained. When the green monkey virus was injected into other nonhuman primate species, different degrees of an AIDS-like illness were produced. Apparently, the strength of the immune response to the pathogen varies in different species. Some are able to harness it more successfully than others.

Some reports suggest that the virus may have entered humans from African green monkeys. Several factors have been implicated which might have led to transmission. The risks include: keeping the green monkey as a pet, sustaining a monkey bite, eating monkey flesh, or rituals involving the injection of monkey blood.

In 1973, Kashamura[1] published the results of his anthropological study of the sexual practices of the people who lived in the Great Lakes area of Africa. His investigations had nothing to do with the AIDS problem, since the virus was not recognized at that time. The author states, "To stimulate a man or a woman and induce them to intense sexual activity, male monkey blood (for a man) or she-monkey blood (for a woman) was directly inoculated in the pubic area and also into the thighs and back . . ."

It is possible that a series of mutations occurred which allowed the monkey virus to cross species barriers. Mutated viruses are usually very toxic to their new hosts. Could the original monkey virus have been responsible for decimating whole populations in the past? Involved scientists are taking sides on the issue. Some say that the biologic gap between monkey and man is too great to allow transmission. Others point to the molecular similarities of some monkey viruses and HIV.[2,3]

Determining the origin of the virus can yield much more than historic interest. If the genetic composition of the progenitor is known, it could be useful for the preparation of a safe vaccine. A vaccine is the major hope to curtail the spread of HIV, which has become a worldwide phenomenon in a short time. The first case was reported in the United States in 1981.

Originally, Haiti was prominently associated with the AIDS disease. It was believed that it spread to the island country by vacationing homosexuals from the United States. However, extensive investigations have shown that the usual risk factors for the disease are not linked to most Haitian patients. Instead, the spread of the virus in Haiti is attributed mostly to nonsterile, contaminated needles. It is the custom in this underdeveloped country to medicate patients by means of intramuscular injections of various drugs. Injections are given for a variety of complaints, ranging from minor headaches to major diseases. Lay injectionists can administer antibiotics and vitamins for nonspecific symptoms. The needles and syringes are usually reused without proper sterilization. It is believed that they became a prominent vehicle for the spread of AIDS in Haiti.

Dysfunctions Due to HIV

The normal ratio of helper T cells to suppressor T lymphocytes (T_H:T_s) in the blood is approximately 2:1. In AIDS patients, where T_H cells are destroyed, the ratio is reversed. Suppressor T cells (T_s) have the upper hand. They tolerate foreign invaders and cancer, always suppressing any immune reaction that may be mounted.

The loss of T_H cells makes the victim susceptible to infections by organisms that are naturally present in our environment, but are usually contained by a healthy immune apparatus. When the rogues are unchecked, they take advantage of the opportunity afforded by the crippled immune system to run rampant, and propagate without restraint. They have earned the name "opportunistic infections." The host that nurtures them becomes gaunt and wasted, and is eventually destroyed. In Africa, AIDS has become known as "slim disease." Several varieties of cancer may also develop in immunosuppressed patients. The advent of HIV has reinforced our appreciation of the enormous job the immune system does in holding potential troublemakers at bay. It is a security that we usually take for granted.

Destruction of the immune system is bad enough. However, this is a mere pittance for the voracious HIV virus. In addition to destroying immune cells, it can also attack the nervous system, eventually demolishing the brain and spinal cord. The virus can be seen inside of macrophages that are located in the brain. The infected mobile immune cells carry their payloads here, causing encephalitis, an inflammation of the brain. This can lead to depression, headaches, memory loss, inability to concentrate, disorientation, seizures, partial paralysis, and dementia. As the brain deteriorates, there is a loss of all humanity. Finally, the disease culminates in death. What an ignominious ending for man, the thinking creature, distinguished from all other organisms! Sometimes, changes in the central nervous system precede the onset of immunologic defects. In these cases, more virus can be isolated from the spinal fluid than from the blood serum. At the time of death, about 70 percent of AIDS patients are demented.

Variants of the virus have been isolated with different genetic structures. There is a correlation between structure and degree of virulence, both in the test tube and in the host. Even in the same individual, the emergence of variants over a period of time has been demonstrated. Progression to severe disease may be related to the sequential appearance of more pathogenic forms.

Opportunistic Infections

The ultimate cause of death in victims of AIDS is uncontrollable opportunistic infections. With the depletion of T_H cells, the central figure in the response, most of the natural defenses of the body are incapacitated. The type of infection depends on the organisms prevalent in the environment. For example, in the United States, the most frequently occurring hostile parasite causes a type of pneumonia called *Pneumocystis carinii* pneumonia (PCP). It is due to a protozoan, a single-celled primitive form of animal life, that lives and divides inside lung cells. PCP occurs naturally in rabbits, dogs, cats, rats, and mice, but usually without causing serious problems. It can spread to immunosuppressed humans by respiratory droplets. An impaired immune system is powerless to contain the parasite, which multiplies unrestrainedly, and is usually responsible for the final death blow. PCP is so common in the immunosuppressed that the diagnosis of AIDS is frequently established only after it is found. The infection always recurs, despite the treatment, and it is never permanently eradicated. There is no vaccine to inhibit PCP.

As the AIDS epidemic escalates, tuberculosis is becoming increasingly prevalent in the United States. It is concentrated in the HIV-infected population, where it attacks many parts of the body, not only the lungs.

In Africa, PCP is not the most common opportunist. Instead, aggressive herpes infections are prevalent, as well as oral thrush, tuberculosis, and diarrhea with severe weight loss. The immunosuppressed are taken advantage of by all sorts of lowly life forms, such as fungi, a bacteria that causes tuberculosis in birds, and many varieties of protozoa, viruses, and bacteria. The treatments that are available are only temporarily effective. The infections always recur, because the damaged immune system never resumes its job.

Tumors are also a frequent cause of death in many AIDS patients. The most common tumor is aggressive Kaposi's sarcoma. It involves cells of blood vessels in the skin, mouth, and gastrointestinal tract, and shows up as purplish spots or bumps. Other cancers may also develop, such as B-cell lymphomas and tumors of the rectum and mouth.

Since the secondary "opportunistics" are usually the immediate cause of death in AIDS patients, rather than the primary HIV virus, some compassionate physicians chose to list only the terminal pneumonia or brain involvement as the cause of death. This attempt to protect the memory of the victim, and spare family and friends from the burden of shame and stigma, has been challenged. Medically, socially, and economically, the virus continues to create chaos. The impact of this submicroscopic peril on the human race is staggering.

Diagnosis of AIDS

The detection of telltale antibodies in the serum is the major screening technique in use. Although these antibodies are mustered by the body to combat the virus, they do little to contain it; however, they are useful indicators of viral presence. Timing is important in the antibody test, since false-negative results are a possibility at the onset of infection. It can take many weeks for detectable antibodies to appear; 6 to 12 weeks is the average time. This makes early diagnosis difficult.

A new phenomenon resulting from the AIDS threat is the rapidly mushrooming "AIDS-Free Dating" clubs. The tested members feel free to continue with their usual life-styles, rather than reduce risks. However, the test can give participants an unrealistic sense of security, because of the possibility of false-negative results. There may be some who have passed the test, but are unaware of their slow progression to AIDS.

In addition, there are carriers of the virus in the population who show few of the clinical symptoms of AIDS. This may be due to the long incubation period of HIV, which varies in different individuals, and can range from weeks to as long as several years. It is thought that the tricky virus may remain dormant as long as other challenges to the immune system are avoided. Acquiring additional infections, which normally activate T_H cells, may provoke the inactive virus to proliferate. HIV establishes itself best in activated cells. A carrier who is asymptomatic may spread the disease to others.

The test can also give false-positive results, which can have devastating psychological consequences. Although the percentage of inaccurate results is low, the numbers can become significant in large-scale testing.

An alternative test for detecting viral presence involves culturing blood cells outside the body. If they are infected, the virus can be demonstrated. However, growing the virus is a difficult procedure, especially in later stages of the illness. As the bulk of T_H cells that harbor the virus are destroyed, the viral count actually decreases. Also, it is an expensive and time-consuming procedure, that requires 1 to 2 weeks to obtain results. Most clinical laboratories are still not equipped to culture the virus.

Another diagnostic procedure involves direct identification of the virus from blood specimens, even though antibodies are not detectable. The patient's plasma is incubated with a commercially prepared human antibody directed against HIV. If there is complexing, the test is positive and the virus can be singled out. Unfortunately, infected persons may have very little unincorporated, free virus in their body fluids. Techniques are available that can amplify the viral presence, but they are cumbersome. More work is needed before the technique can be used for routine blood screening.

An additional tool for diagnosis involves monoclonal antibodies that are made from hybridomas. These antibodies are used to recognize the different subsets of T lymphocytes. Each of the monoclonals complexes with a specific differentiating marker on the surface membrane of a T cell type. Each is made visible with tags of differently colored chemicals. Counts can be made to determine the diagnostic ratio of $T_H:T_S$. A lowered concentration of T_H is characteristic of the disease.

EXPERIMENTAL TREATMENTS

There is no effective, sure-fire treatment available at the present time that can normalize HIV-infected, deficient immune cells. Attempts have been made to augment the failed immune apparatus with its own products, but the results are not very encouraging. Only transient improvements have been obtained with boosters such as the thymic hormone, thymosin, interleukin-2, interferon, transfusions of lymphocytes, and transplants consisting of thymic tissue, bone marrow cells, and fetal liver cells. The virus has never been eradicated.

Children with AIDS are being sustained temporarily with gamma globulin, a fraction from human blood serum. It is obtained from healthy donors, who have antibodies against the usual pathogens in the environment. It is a passive form of immunity, which must be continuously replenished.

Antiviral drugs, which interfere with viral replication, are also being tried. Here, too, the improvement is short-lived, because the destroyed immune function is never replenished. When the drug therapy must be discontinued due to toxic side effects, HIV can be detected once again. Trials with combinations of antiviral drugs plus natural immunoenhancers are being conducted.

Zidovudine, originally called azidothymidine (AZT), is one of the antiviral drugs that has FDA approval for the treatment of selected AIDS patients. However, it interferes with normally dividing cells, in addition to blocking the assembly of the virus. The bone marrow suffers most as a side effect of the drug. A large percentage of treated patients require multiple blood transfusions to replenish the blood cells that normally stem from the marrow. Marrow function returns when the drug is discontinued.

AZT does not cure AIDS. It never totally eliminates the virus from the body, because it exerts its effects only during the replicating stage. Viruses that are present in a quiescent state remain unaffected.

The potential of colony-stimulating factors (CSFs) is being explored. These are hormones that enhance the growth of bone marrow cells, especially PMNs and macrophages. It is hoped that they will counteract some of the detrimental effects produced by AZT in the marrow. The hormones have become available in unlimited quantities by genetic engineering.

The goal in therapy is to intervene as early as possible. If the AIDS virus can be stomped before it does major damage to the immune apparatus, there may be some hope. At present, only the secondary opportunistic diseases can be treated, but there is no permanent cure for any of them. The infections always return when the treatments must be stopped due to their side effects. The immune system never resumes its job.

PREVENTION

Prevention of AIDS is everyone's hope. This will probably require immunologic manipulation by means of a safe vaccine. Theoretically, a vaccine should neutralize the cunning, unmanageable virus before it takes hold. When a vaccine becomes available, the entire world's population will have to be vaccinated, in order to eliminate the virus from the face of the earth, just as smallpox has been eradicated. But this is easier said than done. The virus presents a formidable problem for vaccine development, since it is variable and differs from one patient to another. It mutates readily, changing faces, which complicates the task of preparing a single effective vaccine against all varieties. To date, more than 100 different forms of the virus have been isolated. Researchers estimate that the mutation rate of HIV is five times greater than the record-holding influenza virus. In order to combat influenza, a new vaccine must be prepared periodically. The task of preparing an HIV vaccine is monumental.

A search is on to locate a basic constituent of the virus, which is needed for the survival of all the different forms. This determinant must be antigenic, so that it will be capable of eliciting an immune response. The hope is that the response will be effective against most of the mutants, when the determinant is prepared as a vaccine. However, even if this were accomplished, future changes in the fickle virus might undermine the already-developed vaccine.

Theoretically, any vaccine which is constructed needs to have a dual purpose. It should protect against free virus particles, as well as whole cells that harbor HIV. The virus may hide inside cells in an inactive form, before replication and dispersal. The whole cell might be transferred through body fluids. If its surface appears normal, a vaccine would not recognize the cell, even though it carries the deadly cargo inside.

Another approach involves blocking the receptors on the surface of cells that enable the virus to gain entrance. An antibody prepared against the receptor would unite with it, closing off the attachment sites. The virus would be turned away. Many different strategies will have to be used to finally outwit this formidable foe.

In the meantime, the government has taken measures to protect the public from the growing health problem. It is mandatory to screen all donated blood for the presence of revealing antibodies. Positive blood is destroyed. In addition, when blood products are prepared, they are treated to inactivate the virus. Before the laws were put into effect, transfusion recipients were at great risk for contracting AIDS. They constituted a significant percentage of the casualties; now, their numbers have dwindled. All donations of body organs and sperm must also be tested before use. These precautions have substantially lowered the number of AIDS cases among medical patients.

Recommendations by CDC (Centers for Disease Control) have been sent to all clinicians for the prevention and control of AIDS. There are policy guidelines for physicians, dentists, and those involved in eye care. All instruments, as well as contact lenses that are used for demonstration purposes, must be sterilized as prescribed. Although the AIDS virus has been found in several body fluids, transmission is known to occur mainly through blood and sexual products. There are no known cases of transmission from tears, saliva, insect bites, or pets.

Until an effective vaccine becomes available, the burden of prevention rests largely with the individual. Those who indulge in hazardous behaviors, such as intravenous drug abuse, risky sexual practices, and prostitution must be encouraged to change their life-styles to avoid further challenges to the immune system. It is important to know that new infections may trigger the replication of dormant HIV. When an infected host cell is activated, the virus seizes the opportunity to increase its numbers, causing progression of the disease. In addition, a large antigenic load results in immune suppression. The immune system needs the support of good nutrition, adequate rest, moderate exercise, avoidance of alcohol and drugs, as well as appropriate management of the stresses of daily life. Well-functioning lymphocytes and accessory cells can help to contain the virus.

Individuals with positive tests must take precautions to avoid transmitting the virus to others. Sexual contact with an AIDS patient, or sharp instruments that are contaminated with his blood, are culprits for transmission. Antibody-positive females should not bear children. If there is a pregnancy, the mother should be advised against breast-feeding to avoid additional transmission of the virus. People who have indulged in risky behavior must exclude themselves from blood donations in order to keep the blood supply safe. Individual counseling can help the victim, as well as lessen his threat to the public.

Autologous blood stockpiling, whereby one's own blood is donated before scheduled surgery, is a safe alternative to random transfusions. The American Association of Blood Banks (AABB) is encouraging the use of self blood, since it is the safest and healthiest blood available to the patient. It eliminates the risk of incompatibilities and the possible transmission of diseases. In the liquid state, the blood can be stored for approximately 1 month. Frozen storage of red blood cells is permitted for up to 7 years, according to the standards of AABB. However, this is a costly procedure.

Education is our most potent weapon at this time to contain the lethal disease. As long as no preventive vaccine is available, understanding AIDS can be more effective in stemming its spread than scientific technology. Widespread public education about transmission and prevention must be aimed at the general population to abort high-risk behaviors. Vulnerable adolescents need to be targeted with aggressive educational campaigns. Understanding the virus can be the first step in preventing its spread. If left unchecked, it has the potential to subdue mankind.

SUMMARY

We are experiencing a novel epidemic, which is spreading worldwide, acquired immunodeficiency syndrome (AIDS). It is successfully defying most scientific strategies of control. The immune system becomes irreversibly collapsed, allowing opportunistic infections to flourish. These are responsible for the inevitable death blow. Death can be caused by an organism that is routinely held in check by anyone with a normal immune mechanism. Usually, it does not even pose a threat. Without immune protection, all kinds of infections and cancers thrive. The culprit that destroys the immune system is a chameleonlike virus that changes faces, so it is able to resist being caught. A vaccine prepared against one form may be ineffective against another.

The virus is passed from person to person mainly by blood, semen, and vaginal secretions. Intravenous drug abusers who share their needles are at greatest risk. Homosexual and bisexual men with many partners are vulnerable. Children of infected parents are frequently born with the disease. There is even a report of breast-feeding as the vehicle for AIDS in an infant.

Several years of experience with AIDS patients indicate that the virus is not transmissible by ordinary household contacts. It cannot be caught from dishes or any other utensils as long as they are not contaminated with blood. Shavers, needles, or scissors pose a threat if they puncture an AIDS patient, and are subsequently used by someone else. Likewise, splashes of blood must be avoided. The virus is fragile outside the body, so it is not dispersed by air, water, food, or touch. No cases of AIDS have ever been reported that can be traced to urine, saliva, feces, or vomit.

As yet, researchers have not come up with any drug or immunotherapy that can totally eliminate the AIDS virus, or repair the immune system. There are some antiviral drugs that can inhibit the multiplication of the virus, but the effect is temporary. When the drug is withdrawn, so is its clout. Furthermore, rest periods, away from therapy, are necessary, since the drugs also interfere with normal cellular development. Patients are usually treated for the opportunistic infections and the cancers they develop, secondary to AIDS.

The health departments of many states offer free testing for antibody, which can indicate exposure to the virus. Anonymity is respected to prevent social and economic retaliation. Informational hot lines are also provided. Protocols for protection have been issued to health care workers and other groups that are involved with AIDS patients.

In addition to these preventive measures, our most powerful weapon to stem the spread of this dread disease is public education. Information about behavioral risks is necessary for the public at large, not only for specific groups, since the heterosexual spread is increasing. Also, the general public needs accurate information to help dispel fear and panic about the disease. Vulnerable children, especially, must be made aware of the dangers. An individual's ability to protect himself against the deadly AIDS virus depends on understanding the routes of transmission, the risks for contraction, and how to prevent them. Education is our only effective strategy, as long as science has not produced a vaccine as yet. A fitting slogan that has been adopted by the British is "Don't Die of Ignorance."

1. Kashamura, A. *Famille, sexualite et culture: Essai sur les moeurs sex-*

uelles et les cultures des peuples des Grands Lacs Africains (Paris: Payot, 1973), p. 137.

2. Noireau, F. Orstom, Brazzaville, Congo, Letter to *Lancet,* June 27, 1987, p. 1499.

3. Karpas, A. Origin of the AIDS virus explained? *New Scientist,* 1987, *115,* 67.

9

Recognizing Our Enemies

Arguments are frequently spawned by a lack of understanding. With no facts available, each faction presses for its own opinion. And so it was among immunologists. They took sides on the issue of how antibody specificities are generated against the enormous variety of antigens that the body faces. For many years, the dispute raged fiercely and incessantly, at scientific meetings and in the literature, as long as the mystery remained unsolved.

It seemed unfathomable to many people that the body could contain all the genetic information necessary to code for antibodies against the infinite variety of antigens in the environment. It is estimated that each specific lymphocyte recognizes one of more than a million different antigens. Also, there was no easy explanation to account for the ability of lymphocytes to respond to new pathogens that continuously crop up. New pollutants are being created, and new pesky mutants are evolving. Surely, instructions for lymphocytes to recognize future antigens could not preexist in the genes. It was not until recently, when advances in molecular biology were made, that the facts concerning antibody diversity emerged, and the mystery was solved.

THEORIES

The arguments date from 1900, when Paul Erhlich published his side-chain theory to explain the presence of antibodies in the blood. It is a selection theory that served as a basis for later theories, although it received much criticism at the time it was introduced.

Ehrlich hypothesized that normal immune cells contain a variety of antibody-like receptors on the surface. A particular receptor selects a specific antigen that is introduced into the body, and combines with it. The combination breaks off from the membrane and enters the circulation. The cell is then stimulated to make more of that receptor which continues to be secreted as freely circulating antibody molecules. He proposed that the ability of genes to code for each of the receptors is inherited through the germ line, from the original combination of sperm and egg, and is passed on through the generations.

Ehrlich's theory was later superseded by the clonal selection theory. It states that each lymphocyte makes only one type of antibody-like receptor. Every lymphocyte in the body is endowed with specific genetic information that enables it to respond selectively to one antigen. The information is present in its genes, the structures that occupy fixed locations on the chromosomes. They code for the receptors. When a matching antigen is introduced into the body, it combines with its receptor on the specific lymphocyte. The consummation stimulates the lymphocyte to enlarge, and then to divide to form a clone. The clone of identical lymphocytes differentiates into plasma cells and memory cells. The plasma cells secrete the different classes of antibodies, all of which respond to the same antigen.

The germ-line adherents presupposed the existence of an enormous number of genes, one that codes for an antibody to respond to every antigen that can possibly be encountered. Only one of these genes becomes activated in a particular lymphocyte. The repository of genes is passed along through the germ line, from generation to generation.

The opposing camp could not accept the hypothesis that so much genetic information preexists in our chromosomes. They proposed the instructive theory. It states that mutations, which occur randomly during a lifetime, are responsible for the vast number of antibodies that are produced.

The theory proposed that only a small number of genes exist in the body to code for antibody protein. When an antigen enters a lymphocyte, it serves as a template over which the antibody protein folds. The antibody is molded into a complementary configuration to fit the antigen exactly. Antibodies are then secreted, whereas the antigens are retained for continued antibody synthesis. According to the theory, each B lymphocyte is provoked into generating diverse antibodies, in response to the particular antigens it meets. Antibody diversity continues throughout life, and is propagated anew in the lymphocytes of each individual. The diversity which is acquired is not inherited through the germ line.

Most of the instructive theory is incompatible with modern-day knowledge. Today, we know that proteins are coded for by genes. They are never formed from imprints or templates, and antibodies are proteins. Also, antigens that stimulate the formation of antibodies do not enter into B lymphocytes. The theory was soon discarded.

However, now that the facts have become known, and the mystery that baffled immunologists has unfolded, it proves once again that the middle road is still the safest one to tread. Extremes rarely pay off, even in scientific arguments. The true story contains elements of both theories.

It has been demonstrated that there is a certain amount of genic information in the chromosomes for antibody production, but not one gene for each antibody that responds to an antigen, as was postulated by the early germ-line camp. A limited number of genes is inherited through the germ cells: the sperm and egg. However, this information is manipulated by body cells, the B lymphocytes. During the life of an individual, as his B cells mature, segments of B-cell genes are moved about, forming different combinations and associations. The millions of genic combinations that are possible determine the number of antibody types that can be coded for by B cells. A huge variety of antibodies can be generated from a limited number of germ-line genes. The juggling of genes within each B cell enables it to respond to only one of the numerous antigens that the body encounters.

The Nobel prize in physiology and medicine was awarded in 1987 to Dr. S. Tonegawa for the discovery of how genes that code for antibodies are juggled. He determined that we are endowed with variable genes (V), joining genes (J), diversity genes (D), and constant region genes (C) for each immunoglobulin class. They are passed on from generation to generation, via the germ cells, the sperm and egg. Since there are multiple forms of the V, J, and D gene segments, there is a choice in each B lymphocyte as to which will unite. A single V can join with one of several Js and one of several Ds. The same V can be used again to join with another J and D. The various segments can link together in more than a million different combinations. A limited number of gene segments are juggled about, and combined in different ways, to code for the large variety of antibodies needed. When the stimulated B cell differentiates into the plasma cell, it utilizes only the limited information required for encoding one antibody. All the other information for antibody coding is removed. One of each of the V, J, D, and C regions of the chromosome become combined into one unique piece. Completed recombinations are evident in differentiated plasma cells. These have been observed and recorded with the electron microscope. In comparison, the undifferentiated cells of the embryo show no such rearrangements, since shuffling has not yet occurred. The gene fragments, which have the potential for encoding antibodies, exist separately early in development, far apart on the chromosome, rather than in close proximity. This is the inherited germ-line arrangement. The recombination events occur later on in development, in those cells that are committed to become B lymphocytes. The rearrangements take place in body cells during the life of the individual, rather than in germ cells. Several techniques have been used to verify and demonstrate the shuffling of genes in B cells to attain antibody diversity.

Nature has created this remarkably clever and intricate method for meeting the challenge of our enemies, while using a minimum of genic material. A few immunoglobulin genes have a large combinatorial capacity to generate a pool of diverse antibodies that conform to the great variety of antigens encountered. Genic translocation in a body cell is a means of conserving genic material obtained from germ-line cells.

The threat from newly introduced antigens that never existed before can also be met by this flexible system of rearranged genes. The ability to create the proper alignments that code for antibodies against new assailants can influence survival. The gene rearrangements of one individual may be able to respond more effectively to a particular antigen than those of another. Each of us does better against some invaders than others. This conforms to the rule of nature which is natural selection and survival of the fittest.

Adherents of each of the opposing sides of the argument about the source of antibody diversity have been proven to be partially correct and partially wrong. A few elements of each of their theories fit the facts. Some of the information for antibody production is predetermined in the germ cells. However, this germ-line information is manipulated and expanded in a body cell to create diversity.

The shuffling of genes within body cells can help to explain the lack of concordance which is frequently encountered in identical twins in relation to susceptibility to certain diseases. One twin may develop a disease that is associated with particular genes while the other does not, even though their genes are identical. The twins may not be immunologically equivalent, due to germ line rearrangements that take place in lymphocytes during early development. The juggling of genes in a body cell contributes to diversity in immune potential.

SUMMARY

The mystery that was originally associated with antibody genes is due to the huge diversity of proteins they encode. Anyone who was anybody took a crack at solving the puzzle. For many years, the sparks were flying. Extreme models were proposed, and sides were taken.

It wasn't until the advent of the modern technologies of molecular biology that the true facts about the shuffling of genes were revealed. All factions were proven to be a little bit right, which lessened the tensions. Now, the old hostilities have been forgotten, and there is unity once more, as everyone has the singular purpose of forging ahead. There are still so many questions about the workings of our immune mechanism that require answers. Understanding how nature has designed this intricate system, and discovering all the products it uses, can give us potent weapons to improve health, fight disease, and increase life span.

Our challenge is to learn how to assist and augment the immune system, in order to tip the scales in our favor. Now that we are able to isolate genes, and manufacture their products in large quantities by genetic engineering, the potential of immunology appears to be boundless.

Selected Readings

Textbooks

Benjamini, E., & Leskowitz, S. *Immunology, a short course.* New York, Alan R. Liss, 1988.

Golub, E. S. *Immunology: A Synthesis.* Sunderland, MA., Sinauer Ass., Inc., 1987.

Hanson, L. A., & Wigzell, H. *Immunology.* Boston, MA., Butterworths, 1985.

Kimball, J. W. *Introduction to immunology.* New York, Macmillan, 1986.

Sell, S. *Basic immunology.* New York, Elsevier, 1987.

Journal Articles

Biggar, R. J. The AIDS problem in Africa. *Lancet,* 1986, 1, 79–82.

Bohn, M. C., et al. Adrenal medulla grafts enhance recovery of striatal dopaminergic fibers. *Science,* 1987, *237,* 913–916.

Cohen, L. A. Diet and Cancer. *Scientific American,* (November) 1987, *257,* 42–48.

Council on Scientific Affairs: Vitamin preparations as dietary supplements and as therapeutic agents. JAMA, 1987, *257,* 1929–1936.

Epstein, J. S., et al. Antibodies reactive with HTLV-III found in freezer-banked sera from children in West Africa. 25th Interscience Conference on Antimicrobial Agents and Chemotherapy, Minneapolis, Sept. 29–Oct. 2, 1985, Abstract 217.

Fine, A. Transplantation in the central nervous system. *Scientific American,* (August) 1986, *255,* 52–58B.

Gale, R. P. Immediate medical consequences of nuclear accidents. *JAMA,* 1987, *258,* 625–628.

Graus, F., et al. Sensory neuronopathy and small cell lung cancer. *American Journal Medicine,* 1986, *80,* 45–52.

Haugen, R. K., & Hill, G. E. A large-scale autologous blood program in a community hospital. *JAMA,* 1987, *257,* 1211–1214.

Hayes, B. F., et al. Emergence of suppressor cells of immunoglobulin synthesis during acute Epstein-Barr virus-induced infectious mononucleosis. *Journal Immunology* 1979, *123,* 2095–2101.

Kanki, P. J., et al. Isolation of T-lymphotropic retrovirus related to HTLV-III/LAV from wild-caught African green monkeys. *Science,* 1985, *230,* 951–954.

Kerr, R. A. Winds, pollutants drive ozone hole. *Science,* 1987, *238,* 156–158.

Kessler, H., et al. Diagnosis of human immunodeficiency virus infection in seronegative homosexuals presenting with an acute viral syndrome. *JAMA,* 1987, *258,* 1196–1199.

Khalsa, D. S. Stress-related illness. *Postgraduate Medicine,* 1985, *78,* 217–221.

Koenig, R. E., et al. Prevalence of antibodies to the human immunodeficiency virus in Dominicans and Haitians in the Dominican Republic. *JAMA,* 1987, *257,* 631–634.

Koyanagi, Y., et al. Dual infection of the central nervous system by AIDS viruses with distinct cellular tropisms. *Science,* 1987, *236,* 819–822.

Leder, P. Genetic control of immunoglobulin production. *Hospital Practice,* (February) 1983, 73–82.

Linnemann, R. E. Soviet medical response to the Chernobyl nuclear accident. *JAMA,* 1987, *258,* 637–643.

Longley, S., et al. Familial exercise-induced anaphylaxis. *Annals Allergy,* 1987, *58,* 257–259.

MacGregor, R. R. Alcohol and immune defense. *JAMA,* 1986, *256,* 1474–1479.

Madrazo. I. Transplantation of fetal substantia nigra and adrenal medulla to the caudate nucleus in two patients with Parkinson's disease. *New England Journal of Medicine,* 1988, *318,* 51.

Marlink, R. G., & Essex, M. Africa and the biology of human immunodeficiency virus. *JAMA,* 1987, *257,* 2632–3.

Mayer, C. C. et al. Biologic features of HIV-I that correlate with virulence in the host. *Science,* 1988, *240,* 80–82.

Nash, H. L. Can exercise make us immune to disease? *Sportsmedicine,* 1986, *14,* 250–253.

Nkowane, B. M., et al. Vaccine-associated paralytic poliomyelitis. United States: 1973 through 1984. *JAMA,* 1987, *257,* 1335–1340.

Perry, W. J. Hypothesis that HIV originated in African monkeys is scorned. *Internal Medicine News* 1987, *20* (24):1.

Quinn, T. C., et al. Serologic and immunologic studies in patients with AIDS in North America and Africa. JAMA, 1987, *257,* 2617–2621.

Real, F. X., et al. Steroid-related development of Kaposi's sarcoma in a homosexual man with Burkitt's lymphoma. *American Journal of Medicine,* 1986, *80,* 119–122.

Redfield, R. R. The etiology and epidemiology of HTLV-III

related disease. The Abbott Diagnostics HTLV-III Education Series, 1986, 1–12.

Risenberg, D. E. Can mind affect defenses against disease? Nascent specialty offers a host of tantalizing clues. *JAMA,* 1986, *256,* 313–317.

Rosenberg, S. A., et al. A new approach to the adoptive immunotherapy of cancer with tumor-infiltrating lymphocytes. *Science,* 1986, *233,* 1318–1321.

Schleifer, S. J., et al. Suppression of lymphocyte stimulation following bereavement. *JAMA,* 1983, *250,* 374–377.

Shephard, R. J. Practical issues in employee fitness programming. *Sportsmedicine,* 1984, *12,* 161–166.

Stolarski, R. S. The Antarctic ozone hole. *Scientific American,* January 1988, *258,* 30–36.

Van de Perre, P., et al. Antibody to HTLV-III in blood donors in Central Africa. *Lancet,* 1985, *1,* 336–337.

Virgin, H. W. IV. and Unanue, E. R. Suppression of the immune response to Listeria moncytogenes. *Journal of Immunology,* 1984, *133,* 104–109.

Warren, S. L. Interferon review and clinical experience. *Immunology & Allergy Practice,* 1986, *8,* 33–46.

Wasman, I. and Goodnough, L. T. Autologous blood donation for elective surgery. *JAMA,* 1987, *258,* 3135–3137.

Watson, R. R. Nutrition and immunity. *Contemporary Nutrition,* 1981, *6,* no. 5.

Williamson, W. A., and Greenwood, B. M. Impairment of the immune response to vaccination after acute malaria. *Lancet,* 1978, *1,* 1328–9.

Young, J. D. and Cohn, Z. A. How killer cells kill. *Scientific American,* (January) 1988, *258,* 38–44.

Glossary

AIDS. Acquired Immunodeficiency Syndrome. An immunosuppression due to human immunodeficiency virus (HIV) infection.

Allergy. An exaggerated immune reactivity, or a hypersensitivity to an antigen.

Antibodies. Proteins that are produced in response to an antigen, and can specifically combine with the antigen. They are also called immunoglobulins (Ig).

Antigen. A substance that induces an immune response in an animal.

Autoimmune Diseases. Immune reactions against the body's own tissues, as if they were foreign antigens.

Autologous. Derived from the same individual.

B Cells (B Lymphocytes). Cells which have receptors for antigens, and are capable of developing into plasma cells that secrete antibody.

Basophils. Circulating blood leukocytes that contain granules capable of mediating allergic reactions.

Blocking Antibody. An antibody which interferes with an immune response.

Cell-Mediated Immunity (CMI). Protection due to sensitized T lymphocytes.

Clone. A group of genetically identical cells that descend from a single cell.

Colony-Stimulating Factors (CSFs). Proteins which stimulate the growth and differentiation of bone marrow cells, especially PMNs and macrophages.

Complement (C). Serum proteins that are activated by certain Ag-Ab complexes to produce biologically active components.

Corticosteroids. Hormones from the adrenal gland which are immunosuppressive.

Cross-Reaction. The reaction of an antibody with an antigen, different from the one that induced it, due to shared antigenic determinants.

Graft-versus-Host (GvH) Reaction. An immune reaction in which the grafted donor cells reject the incompatible, immunosuppressed host.

Humoral Immunity. Protection due to circulating antibodies.

Hybridoma. A clone of cells formed from the fusion of a B lymphocyte and a plasma cell which produces monoclonal antibodies.

IgA. The predominant antibody in secretions.

IgD. An antibody which serves as a receptor on the surface of B lymphocytes.

IgE. An antibody which becomes fixed to mast cells and basophils and is involved in allergic reactions.

IgG. Most prevalent antibody in serum.

IgM. First antibody class that is produced against most antigens.

Immunoglobulin (Ig). An antibody is an immunoglobulin.

Immunotherapy. The use of products of the immune system to modify disease.

Interferon (IF). Proteins produced by immune cells and virus-infected cells, that protect healthy cells from the spreading virus. They are also used experimentally as anti-cancer agents.

Interleukin-2 (IL-2). A factor produced by T_H cells that stimulates other cells in the immune system.

Lymph. The fluid of the lymphatic system.

Lymph Nodes. Organs of the lymphoid system that filter out antigens.

Lymphocytes. White blood cells that have many different subpopulations.

Lymphokines. Substances produced by sensitized lymphocytes that act on other cells.

Macrophages. Phagocytic, nonspecific accessory cells of the immune response.

Mast Cells. Tissue cells that contain granules which can mediate allergic reactions.

Monoclonal Antibodies. Identical antibody molecules produced by the cells of a clone.

Natural Killer (NK) Cell. Lymphocytes that kill altered body cells without prior sensitization.

Passive Immunity. Transfer of serum that contains antibodies from an immunized individual to one who is not immune.

Phagocytes. Cells that engulf foreign particles.

Plasma Cells. Differentiated cells, derived from B lymphocytes, that synthesize and secrete immunoglobulins.

Polymorphonuclear Leukocytes (PMN). Cells that participate in a nonspecific immune response, also called neutrophils.

Privileged Sites. Locations in the body that are protected from the immune system.

Stem Cell. A precursor cell that can give rise to different cell types.

T Cells (T Lymphocytes). Thymus-derived lymphocytes.

T_D *Lymphocytes.* T cells that secrete lymphokines when sensitized. They activate other components of the immune system.

T_H *Lymphocytes.* Helper cells that cooperate and interact with other lymphocytes.

T_K *Lymphocytes.* Killer or cytolytic cells, capable of killing cells that sensitize them.

T_S *Lymphocytes.* Inhibit an immune reaction.

Thymosin. Hormone from the thymus gland.

Thymus Gland. A lymphoid organ that controls the differentiation of T cells.

Tolerance. Loss of ability to react against a specific antigen.

Tumor-Associated Antigens (TAA). Determinants that are present on tumor cells, but not on normal cells.

Tumor Necrosis Factor (TNF). A protein that kills cancer cells, and is also responsible for the wasting of the body during chronic illnesses.

Vaccine. An attenuated antigen that is used prophylactically to stimulate an immune response to prevent a disease.

Index

173